Growing Stronger, Growing Free

'The journey of recovery from Childhood Sexual Abuse & the hope for healing'

I0223774

A 2nd collection of works by
'Reaching survivors of sexual abuse'
R.S.O.S.A
Founded by Kate Swift

chipmunkapublishing
the mental health publisher

Published by

Chipmunkapublishing

PO Box 6872

Brentwood

Essex CM13 1ZT

United Kingdom

http://www.chipmunkapublishing.com

Cover Illustration   ('Sunflowers' by Nicky Palmer)

Edited by Fran Harvey

ISBN   978-1-84991-876-3

Chipmunkapublishing gratefully acknowledge the support of Arts Council England.

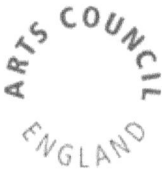

Contributors:

Lela Albert
Carla Robin
Jess Reece
Nicky Palmer
Kate Swift
Veronica Westby
Tori Hollinshead
Wendy Johnson
Karen Dunmore
Patricia Singleton
Meryl Aves
Karen Russell
Ray Redner
Pete Burton
Tasha
Kathy Lloyd-Manning
Linda Rodger
Christina Courtney
Lynn Alston
Veronica Westby
Angelite
Denise Claxton
Michelle Shelley Taylor
Laurie Ann Smith
Michael Skinner
Deb
Sheila Cooper
Jo Descoteaux
Angela Steer
Katrina Pacey
Gemma Merrick

Contributors:

Wendy Lawson
Jessa
Nikki Stone
Ken Doyle
Victoria Barto
Grant Tribemil
Lindsay Greenwood
Shanyn Silinski
Sarah Walker
Mary Gypsy
Janne Helen Tommervåg
Kazzie Kennedy
Mary Calvin
Patty Rase Hobson
Wren Murray
Susan Kingsley Smith
Penny Smith
Kerri Nolte
Sarah Finn
Lorraine Hawkins
Jo R
Fru Hayler
Amy
Ms Rachel E Milano
Cecilia
Ed Shearer
Christopher
Alison Harmer

Dedication

We (R.S.O.S.A) dedicate this book to every survivor of abuse who has yet to find their voice. We have come together in our journey of recovery, helping each other along our paths of discovery.

We wish you restoration and inner peace.

Foreword

A journey of a thousand miles begins with a single step.

This book tells, through poetry, artwork and words, the journey of recovery its contributors are making. Abuse in childhood has profound effects on the abused, often leaving them feeling ashamed; believing that is was their fault; angry; let down; and a whole host of other emotions, as well as leaving them with physical injuries no human being should ever have to experience, let alone a child.

This book is a testimony to the courage, determination and tenacity of survivors of abuse in childhood, survivors that are compelled to live their lives, to be free in spite of their abuse. If you are a survivor, please know *this can happen: you can live your life free of the dreadful trauma you have endured. Remember, you have survived and you can thrive. If you take nothing else from this foreword, please take this.*

I am a survivor myself and these days lucky enough to work as a therapist with survivors of sexual, physical and emotional childhood abuse and those with mental health issues (as some of you will know, there is often a crossover). I count myself as lucky because I am humbled to be the person to hear their story, often for the first time they have spoken of their experiences. Also because some of the most talented, self-aware and beautiful people I have ever met are survivors and thrivers of this travesty perpetrated against children.

Among the survivors I have met there have been artists, writers, teachers, trainers, therapists, accountants, solicitors and many more - childhood abuse has no boundaries, but neither can it stop us fulfilling our potential. We need to take small steps. I often liken the journey to stepping stones: one step at a time. Sometimes we go back, but that's ok - we can take stock and move forward again.

Personally, on my journey these days if I go through a bad patch I know that this is not due to any of my experiences or depression, but that it is down to *life*. I use my coping strategies as best I can and wait for the storm to pass.

Journeys of recovery are as individual as we are. There are no rights or wrongs and what works for one won't necessarily work for another. Listen to yourself, to your own heart and you will know what is right for you. The more we listen to ourselves the easier it becomes.

As well as a practicing Counsellor, I am an Independent Mental Health Advocate and a trainer raising awareness of the effects of abuse and mental health stigma and discrimination.

Carla Robin

Introduction

In our first group book *Silent No More* (published by Chipmunka, 2011) over 90 survivors of childhood sexual abuse came together. We shared the horror and pain of this most horrendous crime. We also shared our hope for healing and some healing inspiration with you. In this, our 2nd group book, we have come together once again to share what it takes to survive. Not only to survive, but to go on and overcome the many obstacles in our path as we live our daily lives.

With the same honesty and poignancy as *Silent No More*, the words on these pages come directly from the hearts of those living with the legacy of childhood sexual abuse. This is not a 'quick-fix' book of solutions; I wish we could all have one of those. Personally I believe that 'recovery' from C.S.A is a journey, and the destination is not an obvious one. I believe it is about taking little steps towards a greater goal, whatever yours may be. One of the most healing things I can do is look back and see where I was 5, 10, 15 years ago... and the look at where I am today. I think 'Tori Hollinshead' sums it up really well: "Recovery is a damn hard process, with bad days at times far outweighing the good times - however, perseverance is the key to any recovery story. Keep at it, because there will come a time when the good days last longer & the bad days become fewer."

It is the moments when you realise something was easier, something was more manageable or that something didn't hurt as much as it once did. It is about turning our 'mountains' into mole hills. It takes sheer determination and the right help and support to keep you on this journey of recovery. In the pages of this book, we wanted to share with you our own struggles and achievements on that same road. We hope that our words and art work will perhaps inspire you, give you some hope and maybe light the way forward if you're feeling lost.

Kate Swift

Please note:

All references to religious beliefs are that of the individual person expressing them and not a shared view of the group. Whilst this book is primarily focusing on the healing journey, the subject matter of some of the content may be distressing. It is possible it may trigger strong feelings, memories, or even flashbacks of your own abuse. It is important to care for yourself as you read through our book. If you find yourself feeling overwhelmed or too upset by what you are reading, please stop and use your support system to help you through your feelings. This is not intended to be a textbook or blueprint for your own recovery... however it is fully intended to inspire you and to give you some ideas of steps you might want to take in your own journey. We strongly advise you discuss any new direction you want to take with trusted friends and/ or professionals.

Growing Stronger...Growing Free...

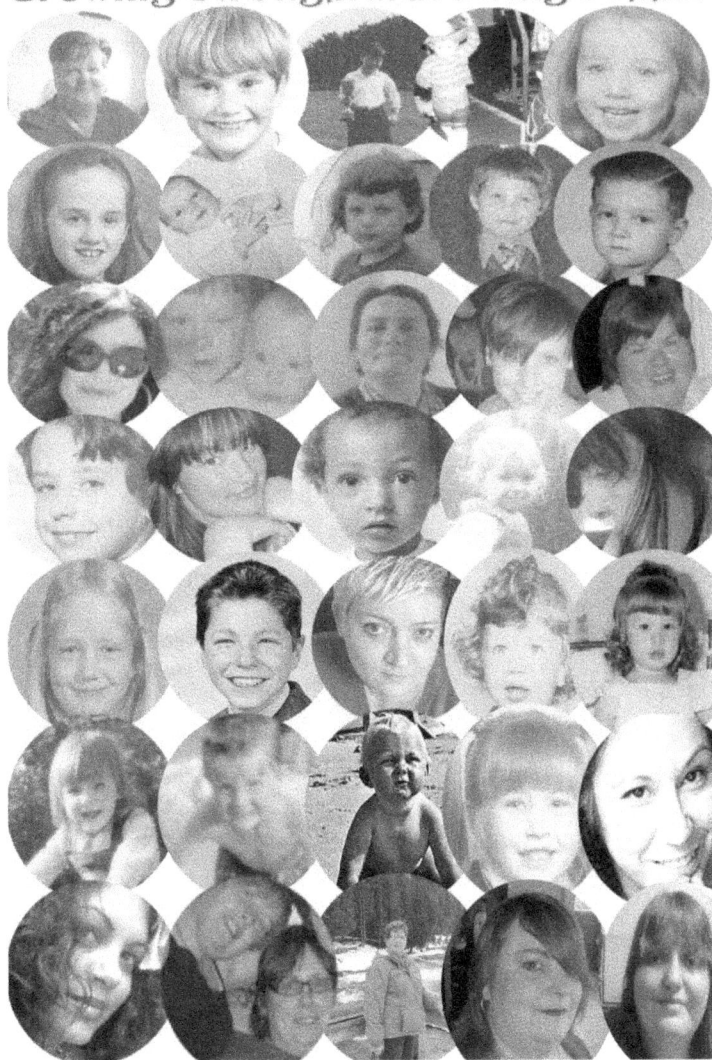

Lela * Carl * Chris * Janne-Helen * Katrina *
Natasha * Alex * Karen * Ed * Michael
Mary * Lorraine & Nikki * Linda * Marie * Tori
Jan * Catherine * Niamh * Penny * Lisa-Jane
Laurie * Andy * Nicky * Simon * Honey
Kate * James * Wren * Cecilia * Pamela
Rachel * Wendy & Angela * Linda * Ronni * Marie

GROWING STRONGER, GROWING FREE

At 'This Tangled Web' people are growing stronger
growing free,
Coming into blossom like a magnolia or cherry tree.
Survivors a many trying to set themselves free
Each and every one had tears, heartache and pain they
have carried thus far.
But at 'This Tangled Web' they see the door open ajar, a
little light far away.
So the tears, heartache and pain start to get whittled
away, happiness starts to return and they go on from
day to day
Start to live their lives and play.

Christopher

Recovery, Working on Me

It was a long road,
Took me time to see where I was going.

It's a lot of hard work,
One day at a time.

I had my ups and my downs,
Some good days, not so good days.

I learn a lot about myself,
The good, bad, and ugly.

Truly amazed how much
I have recovered today.

Never to be the same,
Free to be me.

Lela Albert

Reflections on Recovery

My favourite definition of 'recovery' is: "the regaining of or possibility of regaining something lost or taken away".
Healing from childhood sexual abuse - any trauma, really - is not guaranteed, but the *possibility* is. It is that possibility, that glimmer of hope in the deep, anguished darkness that keeps us moving forward to recover a life that has been stolen.

People sometimes talk about recovery as though it were a static thing, a one-time event that occurs, passes, and is then complete. Recovery, however, is a dynamic process that flexes, expands, and changes as an individual grows. It is a life-long effort because the wounds from abuse are, in many ways, everlasting.

Daunting, isn't it? To think that you will be working at something forever, that it will always be a work in progress. The way we perceive the process will determine how rough the path will be. View it as insurmountable, as though you were Sisyphus himself, doomed to toil hopelessly for all eternity, then you will be unable to sustain the motivation and energy required for you to embrace recovery. If you can fathom, instead, that we are creatures possessing the complex task of growing and developing - regardless of our past experiences - then it becomes a natural part of our daily effort.

Recovery is hard. It is hard but it is *worth* it. All the effort, all the hope, all the blood, sweat and tears, is all worth it because recovery is for you, and *you* are worth it. The responsibility you have to heal your wounds is something no one else can own. It is something that no one else can give you. It belongs to you, and you have a world of possibility with which to regain what was taken away from you so long ago... Yourself.

Jess Reece

Reflections on the Cover Illustration...

'Sunflowers'

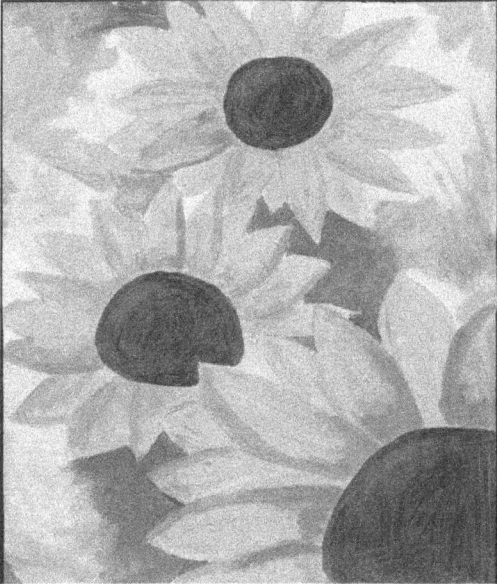

Sunflowers are cool because they just grow and grow beyond everyone's expectations. No gardener can tell exactly how tall a sunflower will grow, how many centimeter boundaries it will break because the stubbornly beautiful creation just won't quit ... like us. We won't quit. We may feel as if we are sometimes, but we're not. We are here. We are alive. Our lives are improving day by day and will continue to do so. We are sunflowers; each and every one of us.

Art & Words by Nicky Palmer

The Sunflower Girl

Have you heard of the sunflower girl?
She stands unique in a field of flowers,
Sunflowers gold, but she's pristine
And even in the bright of day, more radiant than
sunshine in a magical way
Her eyes as deep as the sky above and smile and wit so
readily there,
Such enchantment elsewhere is rare.
Have you known the sunflower girl?
And the way she loves to dance, when the wind winds a
beat through the air?
She lithely twines and twirls and twists; no other like her
could possibly exist.

Sarah Finn

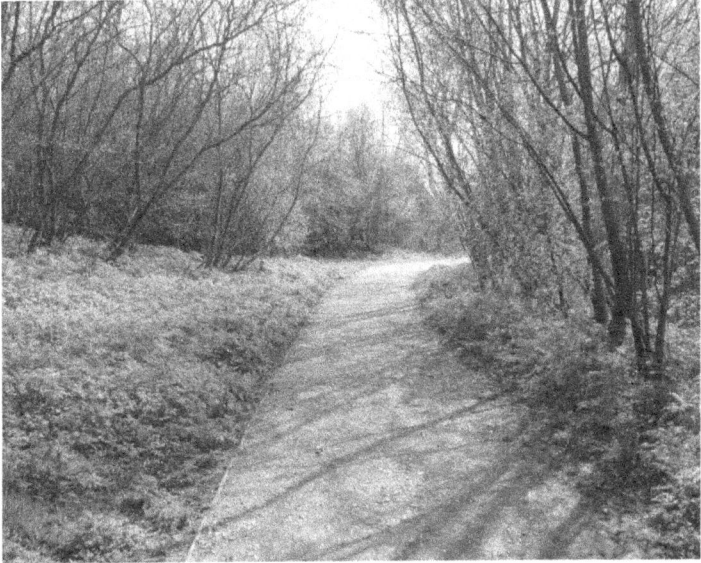

"When I was a child I grew up fearing the world outside.
I remember I
used to think to myself – 'If that is what my family can do
to me,
what is the rest of the world going to do to me?' – but,
you know something,
I learnt that the rest of the world was not such a scary
place
after all; in fact it can be a darn sight nicer than the
place you emerge from as a child."

Words & Photograph by Kate Swift
(Words previously published in *Nobody's Rag Doll,*
2011)

Return to me

Stitching up my skin
Where do I begin?
Healing all the emotional torment
From where you seeped right in
You bled underneath my surface
Tainted all I was
Took me whole and unholy
Then left me scared and lost
I could only see the darkness
I would not see the light
Cradled by my own depression
Long into the night
But now I fully realise
What it means to be free
I will fix my broken wings
And I will return to me.

Nicky Palmer

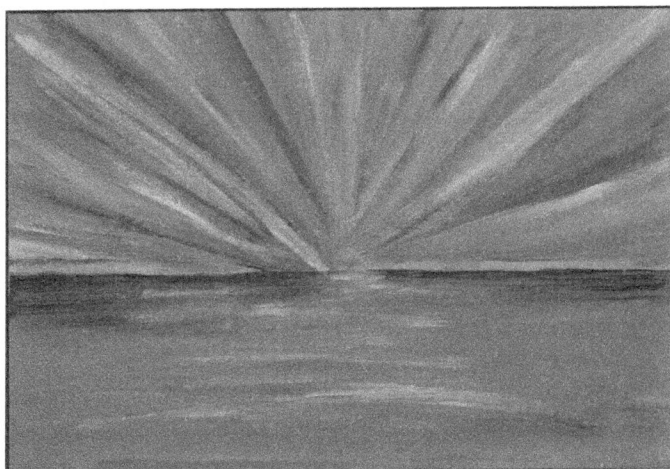

'A New Dawn'

Nicky Palmer

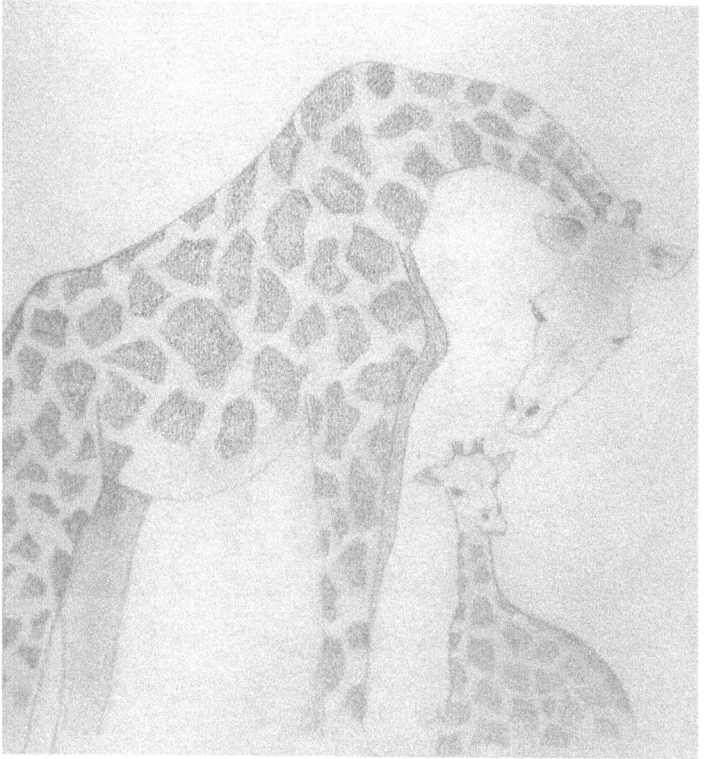

'Motherly Love'

Nicky Palmer

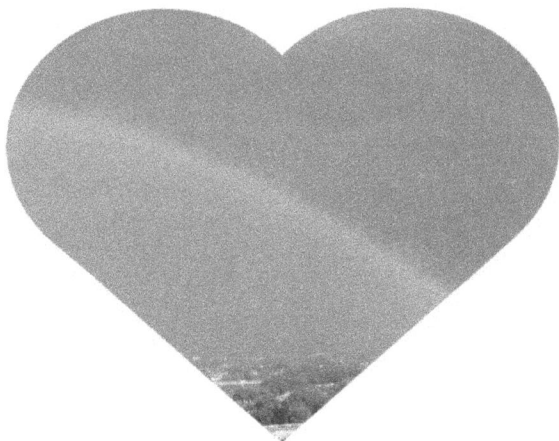

It is time to throw away the old rule book, to kiss the
pain goodbye.

I am done with the history, no time now to sit and
Cry.

With my head held high, I will stand on new and
solid ground.

I am away to chase the rainbows; I know they are
waiting to be found

I have an empty book to fill with memories shiny
and new.

Take my hand and come chase a rainbow too.

Kate Swift
(Previously published in *Nobody's Rag Doll,* 2011)

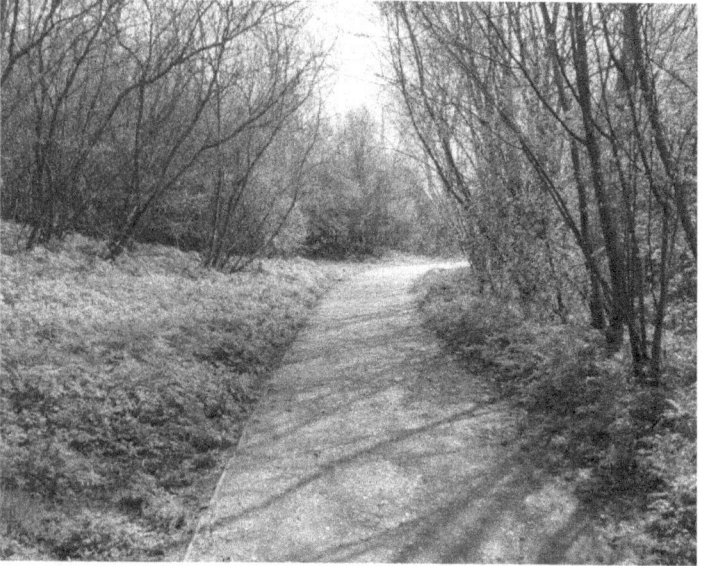

"Every day look in the mirror and smile, because that person smiling back at you is alive and surviving. That person is you!"

Veronica Westby

The Greatest Story Ever Told

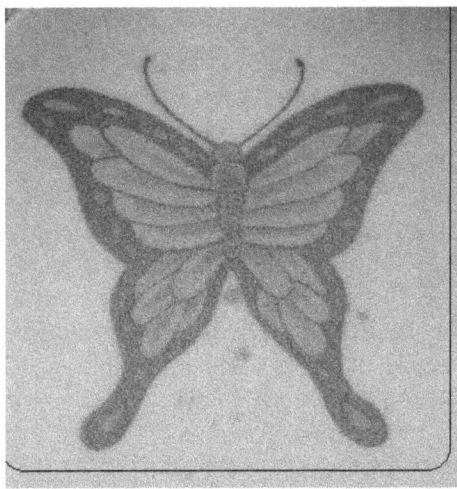

There is a butterfly tattoo on my back. It's symbolic. At the birth of its creation I could not relate, except in my dreams, to this awesome creature. I longed to - I hoped and wished with all my might that I would someday understand the transformation that it was gifted with. For the time being, I turned my two-dimensional piece of art into a 4D creation within me, and from there my journey began.

It took me a long time, too long, in fact, to realise that the chrysalis longing to go through metamorphosis was in fact my broken and wounded mind striving to be restored. When I look back I can now recognise that, and I see how this chrysalis was struggling to survive. It was overdue on the second most important event of its life: life transformation.

I knew there was more out there for me to have. There was life, hope, happiness and a future somewhere full of wondrous things. But I was chained and bound so tightly in my dungeon of pain and suffering that I had given up hope.

I set upon a journey, an unknown, fear-inducing one, having no idea where I would be taken and what would happen to the state of my mind and the battlefield within it. I was very much broken, but yet there was something inside of me, something that would not allow the damaged and broken chrysalis to give in and shrivel away. It seized control on the battlefield of my mind and set about the salvation and restoration process. Various troops joined the battle, fighting for me and willing my chrysalis to restore and develop. Without this army leading the way, the final soldier would not be able to complete Operation Restored.

Some time back the chrysalis started to grow restless and, as the wings began to peek out and stretch themselves straight, the chrysalis seized a bigger control of the battlefield in my mind. Much work was done on the battlefield and at the end of each day, upon contemplation, I began to see the restoration beginning to take place. I admit I was scared. Being healed was unknown territory. I've never been free in the 35 years I have been alive. I have lived my life in a locked steel cage, a cage that I was learning that I had the key to, if only I could find it on the battlefield.

I have a fire in my heart and my 4D butterfly moved from my mind where the battlefield once was to the top of my back. It's resting there for now, wings poised, and is ready to take flight. The butterfly has had an excruciatingly hard journey in its life cycle and sits waiting, with a smile on its face and laughter in its belly, for a soldier to come and help guide it, to break the final chains so that it can be truly free.

Being bound by chains all my life has left me with very little knowledge of how life actually works. I am newborn in a new world, and I need this life explaining to me. Nothing looks familiar. Everything is changed. The colour in my new, restored world is green. Everything is green wherever I look and it is awesome. There are times when the' black fog' will return due to my chemical imbalance, but that's ok, for it is no longer black; it is blue and blue is good. My life will never be the same again.

There is so much more in this life that I ever knew of, there is love, peace and happiness in abundance for those who wish to claim it. Love is changing me, hopes and dreams that I never, ever thought would come true are happening. I never thought that I would smile a true, unblemished smile in my life. I never had until a short while ago. But now I want to smile. I want to laugh. I want to sing from the rooftops. I want to do all these things because I can, and because I have the want and the mindset to do it. I am alive. I am reborn. I am healed. I am survivor through and through! My past has its place in my life, but is no longer ruling my present, which is amazing, and my future is going to be beautiful, more beautiful than I ever dreamt possible. I have been gifted with insight and I am excited, eager, ready and willing to progress. I know there is much laughter to be had and that thrills me and fills me with pure joy.

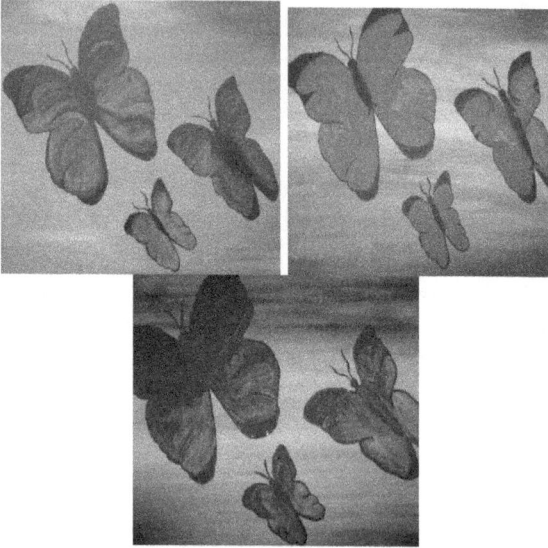

Photo, words and artwork by Nicky Palmer

The day my recovery started...

Sometimes growing up I felt like I was trapped in a world of pain and hate. Very often frustration got the better of me, knowing I'd been threatened not to tell, they blame you if you tell. Getting in trouble at school I so wanted just one person to say, 'it is ok, you can tell'. I never did back then, and when I did I was not believed. I only got away from him when we moved house, or so I thought... I was getting on with my life, had a daughter of my own. One summer day I got her in the buggy and set off for town. I was walking up the road, traffic going by and me proudly pushing my daughter, when I was suddenly very conscious of a car pulling up at the side of me. I went chillingly cold at the sound of a very familiar voice: "Hello you." I spun round, and it was him, he was looking at my daughter. I flipped and screamed, "don't even look at her you don't deserve to live I hope you die; I screamed, you can't hurt me anymore leave me alone". You know I shook from head to foot, but I vented it and felt better... my recovery started that day.

Wendy Johnson

I Believe

To love and believe in yourself,
Is the greatest gift you can give to you,
Picking up the pieces of a broken heart,
Moving forward, releasing the past.

The future is today, the future is tomorrow,
Life is what we make of it,
Scars the reminder of a time gone by,
Healing shows us of a time to come.

I'm looking forward, moving onwards,
My mask removed, my feelings bare,
The future belongs to those who believe,
I WILL BE FREE.

I claim my healing,
I claim my new life,
I am who I am,
I am Strong.

The future is mine and I believe in me.

Karen Dunmore

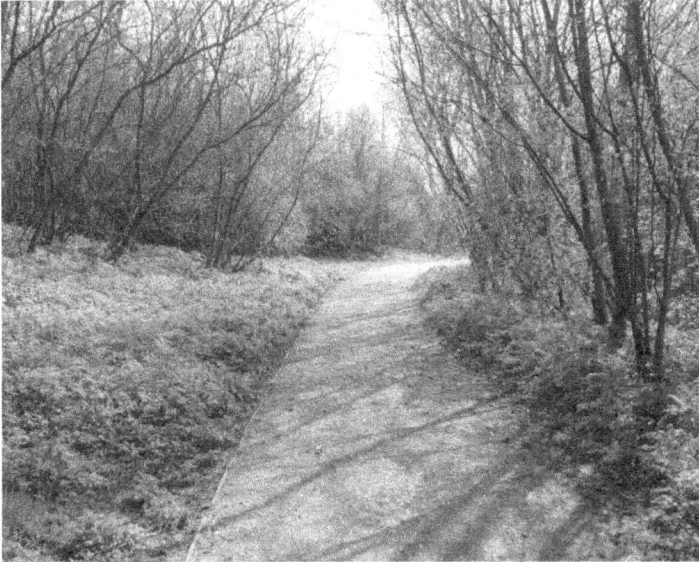

"Recovery is a damn hard process with bad days at times far outweighing the good times – however, perseverance is the key to any recovery story. Keep at it, because there will come a time when the good days last longer and the bad days become fewer."

Tori Hollinshead

From darkness into the light...

As a child I lived in darkness never knowing from
whence I came,
Hiding in a corner full of fear, in constant pain,
My life passed me by in a blur of vile abuse,
I lived in constant darkness & was left feeling I was of
no use,
Then came the day when I had to make a lifetime
choice,
Curl up & die, or stand up & raise your voice,
So to the police I went with my sad tale,
Of this I felt I surely must prevail.
Three years it took to get my abusers into court,
Many times I fell, picked myself up & on I fought,
Justice was served with three guilty verdicts,
This is the result that nobody could predict.
So now here I stand bathed in glorious light,
Having picked myself up & winning my biggest ever
fight,
Recovery has started, the light grows ever brighter,
My name is Tori & I am a born fighter...

Tori Hollinshead

Owning My Personal Power

Owning my personal power is something that I feel like it has taken me years to do. In the beginning, I had no idea what personal power was. If I had any, where was it? What was it? How was it going to change my life?

As a child and a victim of incest, I felt like only my abusers had any power. When I tried to be powerful and not afraid, the abusers quickly made sure that I was put back in my place. I was always afraid of other people - afraid to speak out about the abuse, afraid to speak up and call attention to myself, afraid that if people knew about the incest they would blame me and call me names like trash, whore, or tramp. I was afraid I would die from the shame if others knew. From that position of victim, I couldn't see that I had any power. Those thoughts and beliefs continued into my adulthood.

As a survivor, I had to work hard to discover who I was. Knowing who I was didn't come easy. As a child of incest, I forgot all of that in order to stay sane and to stay alive. I did a lot of trial and error, as a survivor, starting with recognizing the things that I didn't like and didn't want in my life. As a child who saw only negatives from the surrounding adults, how could I possibly, as an adult, automatically know about positives in life? I didn't. All I could connect with, in the beginning, was what I didn't like. After acknowledging and letting go of the negatives for awhile, I could begin to see positive things happening in my life. I could begin to acknowledge:
"Yes, I like this."
"Yes, this feels good."
"Yes, I want this in my life." and finally,
"Yes, I deserve to have this good in my life. I deserve to not have to constantly struggle and be disappointed in myself, others and life in general."

Those changes made room for me to see the positives in my life and in who I was. That change started with learning to love myself and forgiving myself for my reactions to the abuse or to the triggers in life. I could change from reacting to acting which meant letting go of the need for drama and really, fully living my life without the hyper vigilance of my childhood and the stress that went with it. I could find real calmness and peace within myself rather than just the mask of surface calm that most people saw in me.

As a thriver, I am coming into my own power and glorying in it. I am a person of great value. We all are. I am not a victim and I am more than just a survivor.

Owning my own power means I can be me, whoever that is. Shining my Light for everyone to see, loving myself in all of my perfection and imperfections, loving and nurturing all of my inner children while not allowing them to control my adult life, truly loving all of me, even the shadow parts - this is owning my power in all of its fullness. Being able to say 'I am sorry', and then changing any behaviors of mine that have been inappropriate or dysfunctional is a step to owning my personal power. Letting others see me in my imperfections takes courage that I seem to have plenty of. As a child, I didn't think that I was courageous at all. I was. Courage is needed to survive incest. Even more courage is needed to become a survivor and even to thrive, and I am worth it. So are each of you who are reading my words today. I encourage you to look for your own courage. It is there inside of you. Be brave. You can do it. I am no different than any other thriver who has been through the fires of incest and has come out the other side.

Patricia Singleton
You can check out Patricia's Blog @
http://patriciasingleton.blogspot.com

Pure Oxygen

Recently as I was signing out of Facebook, I made the following comment in our survivors support group: 'Sometimes survivors are like pure oxygen to me.' I said it in a heartbeat and have spent time since thinking it over, and my conclusion is how true this is! I remember the first time I *knowingly* met with other survivors... hearing the other stories was difficult and yet just knowing they knew a lot of what was making my own self tick was a comfort. With fellow survivors you can say a lot without having to say a lot. You are allowed to feel any which way, and they are the one group of people in my life who have never said *-just get over it- forget it now-stop talking about it-* Why is that? Because they know what it is to live with this kind of past. They understand that we don't have the luxury of being oblivious or choosing to ignore things as those around us can and often do. It is so healing to hear another survivor say something that you have thought or felt for many years but never been able to express. To see another survivor doing really well can give the rest of us hope when we are in need of it. It gives us some energy to fight on because we can see that what they have is possible for us too. To see another survivor struggling makes us want to pick them up and set them on their feet again... because we have been down in the place to which they have fallen. When life is making you feel suffocated, other survivors really are like pure oxygen. I for one am so thankful for each and every one of them. I know my world would be a much more isolated place without them.

Kate Swift

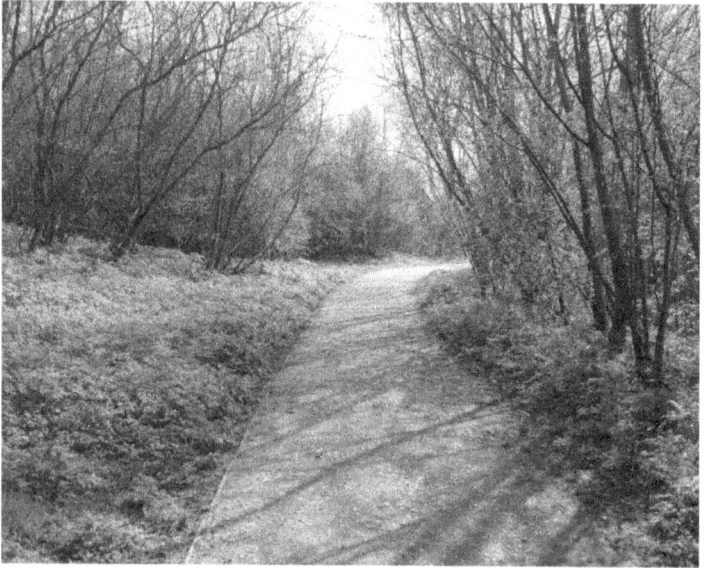

"You know you are recovering when you can look back in time and see a stark difference between you back then and you now."

Nicky Palmer

Recovery
Recovery??? Huh!!!

There have been times when I thought that I had
recovered,
left it all behind, moved on.
Ah, what a relief, I'm whole, healed, got my humour
back.

At other times I've felt that I will never ever recover...
long nights of epic dreams, soaked in sweat, shaking
and terrified,
pain gripping my tissues from the inside
and tugging me back into scenes of brutality.

And then there were moments when I didn't want to
recover
What was the point? Why suffer any more?
If only I hadn't made it - all those years ago.
Standing at the top of the stairs,
holding on to control my trembling
looking down - right down to the bottom
If I closed my eyes and just let myself fall...

Peace was there waiting, tempting me to let myself go.

Sufferers still laugh, smile, joke and say they're fine.
It's crucial to have a 'normal' life
to look normal, have ordinary conversations,
to chuckle at sexist remarks
along with everyone else.

Then the triggers start up again
a word, a smell, sound, image...
anything can start the fear,
set the mind racing,
send the body into crisis,
the horrors immobilizing muscles so that flight is futile.
Just as it was at the time...
the terrible time when it first began.

Recovery is what we aim for,
dream of, work hard for.
At our strongest moments we send kind messages
to other survivors who are having it tough.
"Be strong," we say, "You can do it,"
"It was hard but I was like you once."

And then suddenly, unexpectedly,
we crumble,
lose our power,
feel we never had it,
hopelessness
makes it impossible
to reach out for help.

Seconds are like hours,
weeks like years
we are all alone
again.

But help does come,
friends do appear,
the sun comes out,
warming us slowly,
carefully.
And our wounded heart
is thirsty for love.

Recovery fluctuates,
just like Earth's rolling seasons.
Every storm passes,
each drought is replenished.
As long as we know
that we're not journeying alone
that our stumbles,
our efforts
help another
then we can call ourselves
SURVIVORS
Forever in recovery.

Meryl Aves

Healing From Abuse Means Doing the Work of Healing

Healing from abuse means doing the work of healing, not just talking about the abuse. Yes, in the beginning of healing, talking about what happened to you is important. In fact, talking, in itself, can be very healing and breaks the bonds of silence that your abusers taught you. At what point in the journey, do some survivors get stuck in the drama of telling their stories and never move beyond that point? How do you tell when you are healing from telling your story and when you are just plain stuck?

For me, I told my story over and over for about 10 years, but that wasn't all that I was doing. I was reading books on healing from incest. I was writing about my own experiences. I talked to other survivors who were doing their own work. I went to two different groups for counseling as well as doing individual work with two counsellors over that ten year period. I also had two 12-Step sponsors that gave me personal work to do on healing from incest.

I did the work of recognizing the lies that my abusers told me. For many survivors, those abusers were one or both of their parents. Exposing the lies of your abusers is a very important part of your early recovery. So is telling your story. Both are healing steps that need to be taken.

Telling your story does not mean creating drama for yourselves or others. Some survivors create drama as a way of recreating what they were used to as children. This is why exposing the lies of your abusers is so important. When you see those beliefs as lies, you can begin to choose how you will react to your triggers, how you will react to the people that, on purpose or accidentally, set off those triggers in you.

I believe that triggers happen to show you where you still need to work on yourselves and the issues behind the triggers. Triggers don't happen to make you blow up all over someone else. When you do that, then you become like your abusers and abuse someone else. That is what was done to you as children and it is what you may continue to do to others until you learn that you don't have to continue those unhealthy patterns of behavior.

A pattern happens when you repeat the same behavior over and over. I have learned to look for patterns in my own behavior. With awareness of patterns, I can then decide to make changes or stay the same. If my behavior is hurting me or others, I decide to change. That in itself is a process that takes time with lots of trial and error and apologies along the way until I change that pattern with a new, healthier pattern.

One example that comes from my own life has to do with anger and rage. Rage is un-healthy anger that grows and grows and gets blown all out of proportion, usually because the first signs of anger were not recognized or were ignored, denied or stuffed deep inside. Rage eventually comes out when the pressure is too great to hold it in any longer. It comes out, usually on someone that totally doesn't deserve it. I used to do this all the time. Anger wasn't allowed in my house except for the rage that my dad carried around so my anger was denied and stuffed with food until the rage came rolling out like hot magma from an out of control volcano damaging everything in its path.

Rage was the first feeling that I learned to deal with, because it was so volatile that I could easily see the damage that I was doing with it. Doing this work isn't a matter of feeling shame for the fact that I couldn't control my rage. Doing this work is a matter of feeling the feelings without allowing them to hurt myself or someone else.

Rather than feeling shame when I get a new awareness, I forgive myself for not seeing the pattern sooner, then I set out to change the situation so that I don't continue to hurt myself or someone else. It isn't enough to feel bad about my behavior. If I am being hurt or someone else is, then I need to change that behavior. If I say I am sorry but continue to do the same destructive pattern, then I am not really sorry. Any behavior that I continue to do, I am getting something out of it or I would quit. Feeling shame or guilt about a behavior is a sign that change needs to happen. If I know that my reactions are out of proportion to the situation, it is my responsibility to do something to change my reaction. If I am looking to create drama, I will find an excuse to do it.

With healing comes responsibility for my own actions and reactions. Another person does not trigger me. My own issues are what trigger me, not what someone else said or did. Those issues trigger me because I haven't healed that particular issue. It is not anyone else's responsibility to fix me, just as it is not my responsibility to fix anyone else. The triggers will keep coming until I am healed in that area. I am not saying that I am at fault or wrong or bad because I am still being triggered. I am saying that it is my responsibility to heal me so that I am not triggered. It is my responsibility to do my own work to heal. If I am refusing to see the awareness that has come into my life because of my triggers then I am still playing victim. I am still believing my abusers' lies that I am not capable of taking care of myself. Or I am still believing the lie that I am too stupid and that I am worthless and have no value and can't make decisions for my own self. No matter what you said about me or to me, I alone am responsible for what I do with that information. You do not make me angry. I choose whether to get angry or not. My actions are my responsibility. How I respond to a person or a situation is my responsibility, not yours. I can't blame you for what I am feeling. I choose whether I stay stuck in the victim role or I move forward in the survivor role.

Saying that I never meant to hurt someone doesn't mean a thing if I continue to hurt them. Feelings are not inappropriate. It is what we do with them that can be inappropriate. I have no way of knowing what another person is feeling unless they tell me. What I may see as insensitivity or lack of empathy in another person may not be that at all. I cannot know or guess what another person is feeling. What that person may say has nothing to do with me and everything to do with them. I cannot second guess other people unless I am intent on creating drama for myself. If I want to create drama, drama will find me. When I say someone else is insensitive, I am projecting my own insensitivity onto that person.

I want to heal from incest. I do not want to be defined by incest. Incest happened to me but is not who I am. I am a human being living and growing through my experiences. Sharing my experiences does not make me better than you or perfect. I am far from being perfect. I make mistakes. I still sometimes see someone else hurting and out of my feelings of compassion I want to make their way easier. Sometimes I can help. Sometimes I cannot. Sometimes I even manage to make situations worse. Sometimes I play devil's advocate and try to look at the bigger picture. I don't know where the term "devil's advocate" came from. I don't see it as bad. I see it as the simple process of stepping back and looking at more than the immediate view or seeing a different view than everyone else is taking. Being different is not a bad thing.

You have the power to heal yourself. You have to do the work if you want to heal. My question for you is, "Do you want to heal?" or "Do you want to stay stuck in victim mode and blame everybody else for your life?" If you want to heal, at some point, you have to move beyond the blaming stage of healing. In order to heal, at some point in your life, you have to take responsibility for your present and future. Responsibility for the abuse of your childhood belongs with your abuser. Responsibility for what you do with your adult life belongs with you.

Patricia Singleton

You can check out Patricia's Blog @

http://patriciasingleton.blogspot.com

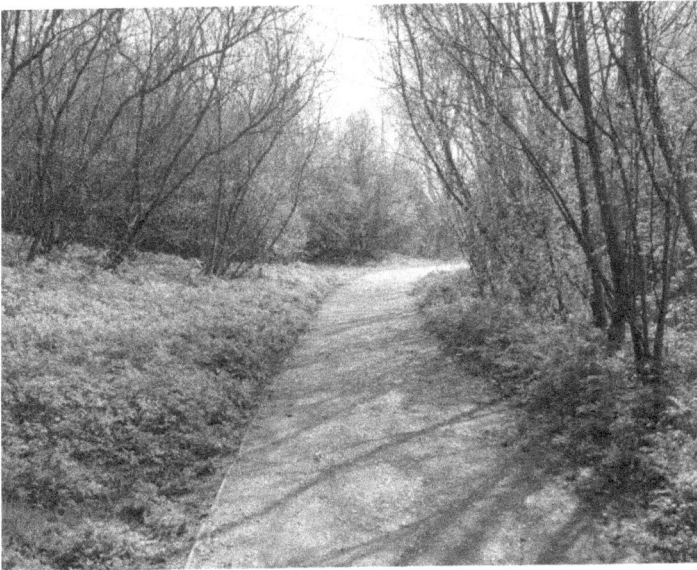

"Feeling a hundred times more confident now. I mean, I don't have to live with dirty little secrets. I don't have any... he does!"

Wendy Johnson

Onwards We Go…

The pathway to your healing stretches out in front of you

You feel so many emotions; the journey seems too hard to do

At first it is hard just to stand again

You feel a deep and wounding pain

You wonder how to put one foot in front of the other one

The journey seems impossible before it has really begun

Yet with time and help you begin to move along

Once feeling so weak you begin to get strong

The path is not easy, sometimes we lose our way and we stumble

Our mind in such a crazy jumble

But onwards we go

And into a survivor we grow

Now we can see in colour and feel a sense of release

The path takes us from our nightmare into peace

The journey has been epic, you never thought you could come this far

From a victim to a survivor, that is what you are.

Kate Swift

I Will Be Strong

I was a little girl
I didn't know right from wrong
I was weak and you were strong

You used your strength to gain my trust
Then abused me as if it were a must
That is not what Daddies do
I now know that this is true

You said you loved me but that can't be fact
Because with my Mother you made a pact
To always lie and never tell
and stay together as if all is well

Well it's not all good, at least not for me
Because I don't know what to do, you see
I must rid myself of this anger and pain
and with that the control I will gain

I know I must, but it's hard to do
Cause only you and I know what you put me through
You said stay quiet and never tell
I say to you just go to 'hell'

It is not me that should carry the shame
It is not me that should take the blame
I will speak out, I have a voice
You can't keep me quiet, you have no choice

I was a little girl
I didn't know right from wrong
But now you are weak and I am strong

Karen Russell

A Phoenix Rising

I am burnt, destroyed
In the fires of hell
My ransom paid
By the blood of another
From the ashes of my soul
Full of Holy Fire
I rise
And streak to the heavens
Reborn I soar
From the loftiest heights
I spy the universe
And greet its endless boundaries with zeal
Nothing will hold me down
I am flame
I am alive
I am...
A Phoenix Rising

Ray Redner

This poem was first published in 2011 in
The Echoes of My Mind and The Voices of My Soul'
also by Ray

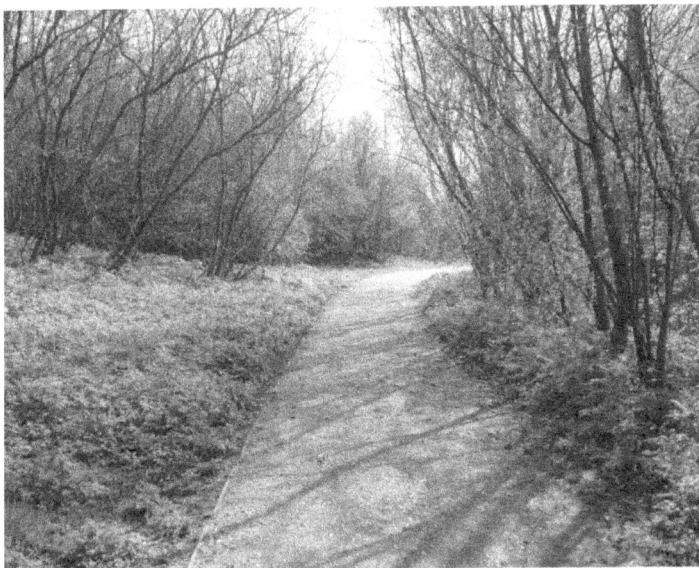

"I am headed over to celebrate recovery and taking my five-year cake to my home group. ...I spent many years being angry and taking it out on me. I am so glad to be clean and sober long enough to be able to start to love me. Some days I don't know what loving me looks like, but today I do. It is celebrating a victory with my friends."

Pamela Abraham

Thoughts on 'Recovery'

Our recovery started when we broke the silence (Our Silence)... Our journey is punctuated with stages of recovery and positive moments... Every point on the road is important... Nobody's achievements can be diminished by a word like 'fixed' - we are not cars, we are people and we are unique as individuals.

Pete Burton

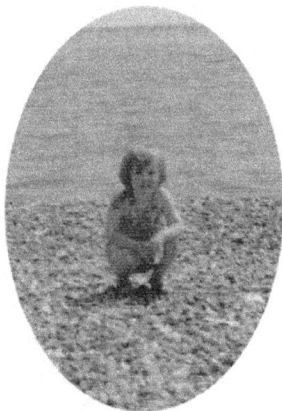

My Journey to Recovery

I'm 'Tasha' and this is my personal account of my journey up until today, 2012, after discovering at the age of 29, almost 11 years ago when I first disclosed my whole life to a very dear psychotherapist in London, who confirmed that I had been sexually abused by my maternal Grandfather. It was the hardest thing I have *ever* done but also *the* best thing I have ever done for *me*.

I had disclosed to a dear friend at the age of 24 and another when I was younger. I told them what had been 'going on'. The way I told them then was as if it was my fault and I wanted to protect him, as he was still alive. The story today is different: I never managed to get him convicted, as I was never at the right place to do so and I was not given the right support by my family... my mother, aunt, uncle all on the maternal side... but I know that I was *not* to blame. I was a child robbed and stripped from all my innocence and inner beauty. I am learning to *love* myself. It is a huge task, *but* I do forgive myself, which to me is a great breakthrough as my sexual abuse went on until I was 22, from the age of 5 or younger.

I get flashbacks and triggers from smells, clothes and toys. I can now reassure myself it is OK, I am safe and they are just a memory and it is not happening now! I take a low-dose anti-depressant - these are my props to get me through the darkest days following a time when I decided that I wanted to end my life - and tried to do so only last year, through overdosing. Luckily I woke up the next day with a very bad head. Since that day I am grateful for the sun, the moon, the clouds, the air I breathe and my family. Most important of all my children, who do not ever deserve to deal with the aftermath that might have been because of some very sick person.

One thing is for sure, I would not have taken my first step to my recovery without the sound advice that my closest friend, who I lived with at the age of 15 (her and her parents) gave me: to go get help. Hence my counselling and, of course, my husband's continuous support love and faith, who has *always* believed in me and puts up with my hostile moods and pushes me out of my comfort zone whenever needed.

I will win this battle because I am in charge of me now. I would like to take this opportunity to thank 'This Tangled Web' for giving me this chance to put my voice out there as it has been silenced for far too long. I have come to know some amazing, strong, beautiful people who prove that where there is hope, there really is a will and also a need for everyone to speak out, unite, be free and understand that the world does have good and people can do good. I look at this journey as ongoing, because that is life, but I live with the hard lessons I have learned and the truth. Now I like to think of myself as a chrysalis that contains a butterfly that will fly free with all the beauty and changes that are before me. The way I see it, the road to recovery is the only road, it's one-way, and sometimes you fall off and get dazed and all you can see is black, but you get back on that one-way road and you carry on driving because you really are worth it! You, we, I survived the worst and that is over forever, and that is a huge accomplishment that deserves a trophy at the end. It is a trophy that I am prepared to pick up for myself (metaphorically speaking).

Tasha

Growing Stronger, Growing Free

I WAS LOST ON MY PATH ONE DAY

YOU SAID 'COME, LET ME SHOW YOU THE WAY'

I HAD BARE FEET ON THAT HARD, STONY GROUND

YOU HELD MY HAND AND SHOWED ME AROUND

I CHOKED ON MY TEARS

WHEN I TOLD YOU MY FEARS

YOU WIPED THEM AWAY

SO TO START A NEW DAY

YOU SAID 'COME, LET THEM GO'

BECAUSE PEOPLE HAD HURT YOU A LONG TIME AGO

I HAD ANGER AND RAGE ~ LIKE I WAS STUCK IN A CAGE

BUT YOU STILL WALKED WITH ME

YOU WERE MY EYES, YOU COULD SEE

I WAS BLEEDING AND TORN

FROM THE BRAMBLE AND THORN

BUT YOU STILL HELD MY HAND

WHEN WE CAME UPON SAND

TO THE LIGHT OF THE SUN ~ YOU SAID GO ON RUN

BE FREE MY FRIEND YOU CAN LEAVE PAIN BEHIND

HOPE, LOVE, JOY AND PEACE YOU WILL FIND.

Kathy Lloyd Manning

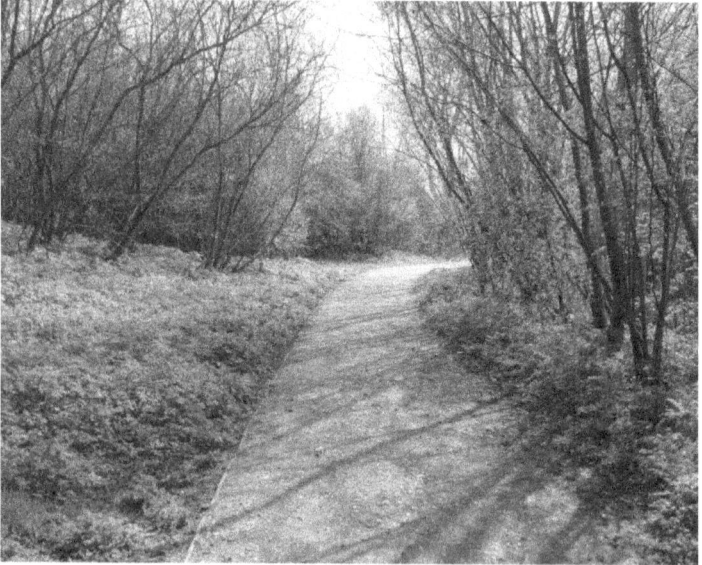

"Every survivor deserves a beautiful dawn... we just need to work to make it happen and believe that we do deserve it."

Kate Swift

Recovery

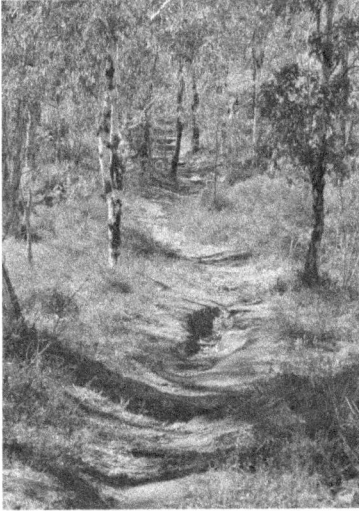

As with any traumatic event, surviving sexual abuse takes time, effort and personal struggle. More often than not it feels like one is endlessly climbing up hill. Whilst I am not a survivor of sexual abuse (I am of physical/emotional abuse) my mother is, and she has shown me that despite the psychological, emotional and physical scars that it leaves behind, a person can overcome those and achieve great things. My mother spent years overcoming her abuse. But she didn't let it hold her back. She has worked to get multiple masters degrees despite having a limited education, and has worked hard at developing other skills. But more importantly, she has used her own experiences to help other survivors through their own recovery.

I think that one of the most important steps in a person's recovery from sexual abuse is their ability to focus their own pain and struggles to support another survivor. That then enables both survivors to continue in their journey to recovery. I encourage all survivors to keep walking that uphill path because the view at the top is beautiful and is well worth all the pain and toil.

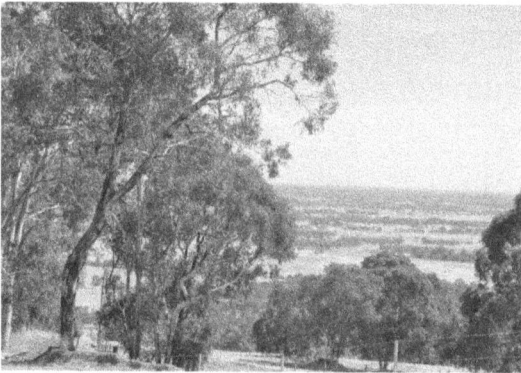

Words and photographs by Ray Redner

Growing Free

When we are little we are in pain,
When we have nothing to gain,
Then when we are older we have a choice,
We give up or go make it better,
It is not easy making it better,
But we feel better, and life matters,
You feel the pain the little one has,
You heal the scars your little one has,
You love yourself like no one did,
You choose to heal and make it better,
You're happy when you heal,
The best you can feel,
The little one is free of all the pain,
When she knows it was not her fault,
And can try and build a life...
The life you never had.

Linda Rodger

My thoughts on healing the pain of abuse

It is never easy to heal from the pain that abused children feel. Who will believe you? is the start. Can you deal with all the pain and the hurt you feel inside? It is not easy, but it's worth the effort to be free from the hate, pain, and worthlessness you feel over what you dealt with the best you could. Do you want to stay with the feeling that you're no good and worth nothing? Or do you feel the need to be free and deal with the pain? It is hard. However, when you find the right therapist and you start to get through the hurt and pain your little one suffered, little by little you start to feel better. The little child of yours can be free and happy. It feels much better when you can choose what you want out of life-the choice you never had before you recovered from the abuse.

Linda Rodger

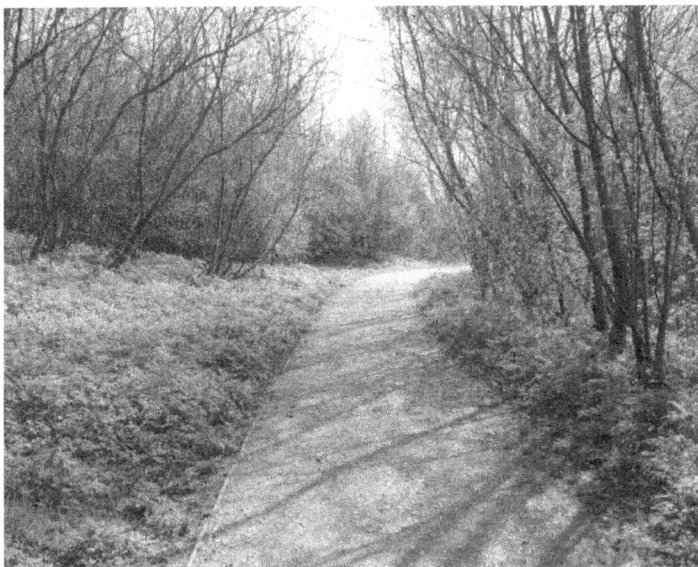

'If you get up one more time than you fall, you will make it through.'

Author unknown

Our Noble Beast

Abi came into my life because I was just back home from yet another failed relationship and suicide attempt. My parents thought it would be good to get me something to focus my attention on and to give me a sense of responsibility, and thus was born the pact that if I got Abi that I was to do no more self-harming or overdoses. I agreed. The consequence was that, if I broke the pact, Abi would be taken to the dogs' home. This was to be the beginning of a very loving relationship and an amazing friendship.

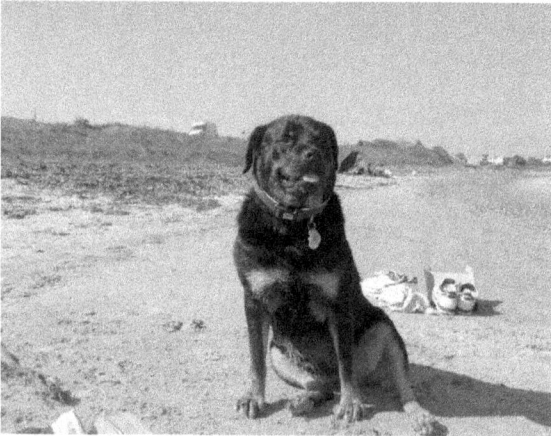

I'd moved back to Northern Ireland and in with my parents, and within a few months so did my abuser, to the very same town. But Abi gave me the confidence to go outside again. She had to be walked and lots of it, and she was a Rottweiler and provided me with the security to go outside.

We used to get up early, around 7am most mornings, and we went away for our walks - me with my headphones in and Abi with her head in the air, ears pinned back.It was almost like Christopher Robin and Winnie the Pooh - we had an instant bond and went everywhere together.

But I digress. These walks took us over the football pitches and down onto the beach where Abi used to pick up big sticks of kelp. Running along the rest of her walk with this in her mouth, she'd bite through it and end up with a wee stump left at the end. We used to joke, saying it was her stogie, sort of like a cigar. We'd continue down along the harbour and across the commons, and back home across the cricket pitches and into the house for breakfast, and then she'd have lay and slept whilst I wrote my journal.

We did everything together and anyone new coming into my life had to meet with Abi's approval. If she didn't like them, she made it clear and she kept me safe and allowed my shattered and battered self confidence to rebuild. Her sheer size and breed made most people back off, and that made me feel secure and protected.

I believe the animal chooses us, not the other way around and in Abi's case this was very, very true. I met her when she was looking for a new home. She was only 6-7 months old, and we grew together. I would have done anything for her and I know the feeling was mutual. Her sudden death shocked me and it was so soul-destroying to know I wouldn't ever see her or walk with her again. It damn near broke me, there will never be another Abi, aka Pumbah.

I never broke my pact with Abi ever, including when she passed away due to complications after knee surgery last year. I remember getting the phone call at 4am in the morning from the on-call vet to say Abi had passed away very suddenly. I dropped the phone and started to sob like a child I couldn't believe my friend, my Pumbah, was gone forever. We went to the vets to see her and she looked so small and I just wanted to pick her up in my arms and hold her forever and never let her go. As she lay there I bent in close and told her she may be gone, but our pact still stood. I wouldn't disrespect her memory by doing anything.

Abi was named after the character in N.C.I.S. She was very like her in nature - all sharp and spiky on the outside, and very soft and cuddly on the inside. Her ashes are on the fireplace and in pride of place. She may be gone from our lives, but she will never be forgotten.

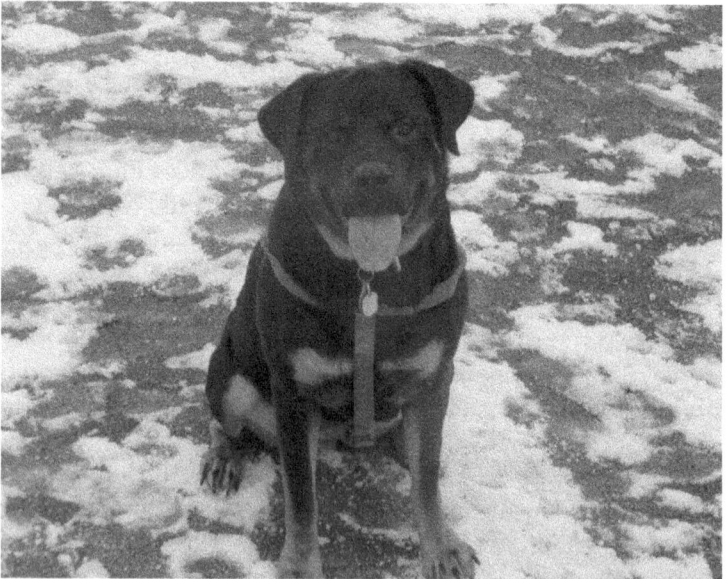

R.I.P. Abi Courtney / Moore – Our noble beast.

Words and photographs by Christina Courtney

Sit With Me

You say you want to help me
But don't really know just how.
Well let me try and tell you
Just be here with me right now.

Sit with me while I'm crying
Or when I'm feeling scared,
Or when I'm feeling all alone
With no one who ever cared

Sit with me while I'm bleeding
From a self inflicted cut
Because I'm very frightened
And am stuck within this rut

Sit with me when I overdose
And I'm fighting off the sleep
Because I really want to die
I feel I'm in too deep

Sit with me and just listen
To why I've ended up this way
And just be there to help me
Through yet another day

Sit with me in the darkness
When I really just can't sleep
And thoughts start running through my head
And in the memories creep

Sit with me and don't judge me
'Cause I need you to understand
That I don't want to be this way,
And just reach out your hand.

Lynn Alston

Friendship

A friend is one who loves you
No matter who you are
Who knows all of your secrets
But never pushes you too far

A friend is one who listens
And who is always there
To offer you a shoulder
And to say that someone cares

A friend is one who is there with you
In good times and in bad
Always there to have a laugh
Or when you're feeling sad

A friend is someone special
To cherish and to hold
Always kept within your heart
Together growing old

A friend is one who is always there
To lend a friendly ear
And friendship that will blossom
As you go from year to year

A friend will not desert you
When things just get you down
They'll cherish you and love you
When all you can do is frown

You've become that friend to me
Been there when it's bad
You have been a rock for me
For which I'm really glad.

Lynn Alston

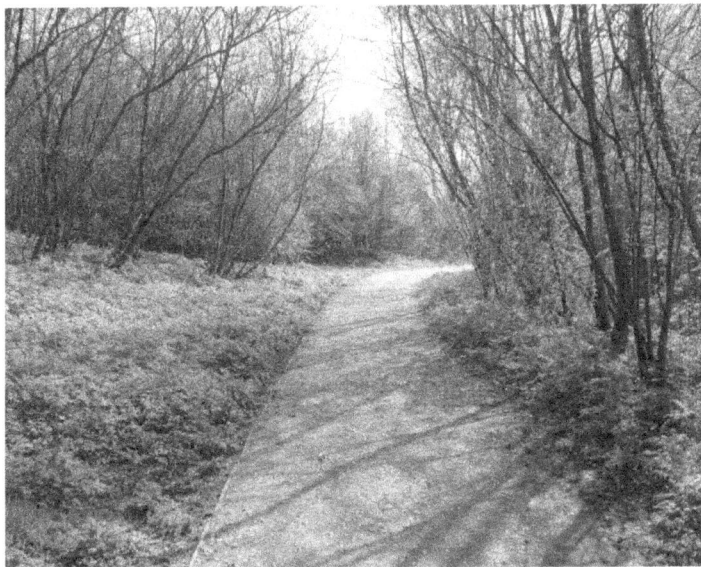

"I really do want to dance in that rain, I'm ready."

Wendy Johnson

Reporting Historical Abuse as Part of My Healing Journey

I am going to write about how I came to a decision to report historical abuse - my historical abuse. By historical abuse, I mean sexual, physical and emotional abuse that I suffered as a child from members of the family. In this article I will be focusing on just one abuser.

Reporting the abuse was not a decision I made easily. In fact, I had thought about it on and off for the past twenty years or so. I am now coming up to my mid-forties. I believe that fear always prevented me from reporting it until now. 'Fear of what?' you may ask. Fear of not being believed; fear of how my own lifestyle will be perceived; fear of what will happen to my own children; fear of repercussions from the offenders and their family members; and, yes, a fear that was installed in me by the mother who was a perpetrator of much of my abuse, fear that if I said anything it would kill her. These are just a few factors of fear that I had, and still at times do have.

So what prompted me to report everything now? One of the biggest things was knowing that I had the support of close friends, and that no matter what they would be standing with me throughout all of this. The key element was that they believed me from the bottom of their hearts. The other important factor was that the mother had now died, so the biggest of my fears was taken out of the equation and I could not ever be blamed for causing her death. I guess, also, my own personal growth and training as a therapist helped me to get to a place emotionally that I could at last speak publicly about what really went on for me as a child. I had finally learnt and believed that I was entitled to have a voice and be heard.

Believing I was allowed to have my voice was paramount throughout this process. I knew I would come across many hurdles where that belief would be tested to the limits, but I had to trust that those that knew me and believed in me were telling the truth when they kept telling me that I am much stronger than I ever allowed myself to believe. The truth of it is that I had survived the abuse firsthand, and therefore, having survived that, telling my story was never going to be as painful as living it in the first place. I also knew now that I had choices and I was no longer that small defenceless little girl who had no way of defending herself. The biggest thing for me was my overriding need and desire to protect other children from encountering the harm that I had received from the hands of my abusers, and this was to be the turning point in my decision to make the report.

It had come to my awareness that one of the abusers had access to children as young as four. As far as I could make out, this access was with only the children present. I didn't know if he had the certification for a criminal records check to ensure that he had no criminal record for any harm to children. Also, the access to these children was in his own home, where the other abusers also lived.

I had also been given information from other family members that he had assaulted at least one other family member when they were a child, and had asked another young family member to get in bed with him.

So with that knowledge, I had to then further explore my own history with him and the impact it had had on me. I looked back in detail on the events that had occurred. I could remember how I was feeling at that time, and the key to me understanding that what had happened wasn't just children exploring their sexuality or, as some may say, playing doctors and nurses, was the knowledge that everything he did to me was done for sexual gratification. This was not innocent children playing, but an adolescent wanting sex. Another key factor was his pressure on me to keep it a secret or I would be in serious trouble. This is a classic action of a predatory offender grooming their victim into silence by making them fear that they are doing wrong, and not vice versa. This is a key factor of why victims of abuse keep the silence and protect their abusers. They have installed in them a huge amount of fear that they are the ones who are doing wrong, and if they tell anyone, they are the ones who will be hurting everybody, including their abusers.

Having explored in my head and heart what this would entail, I then had to think about how I would go about actually reporting it. In that I was fortunate to have had sufficient training in various professions of the care field. I had also received child protection training within my studies as a counsellor, which gave me the basic information of where I would have to go to report these crimes.

I contacted a friend I knew in my local police force and asked if she could visit in a professional capacity, as I needed some advice and guidance. She visited along with a colleague of hers. This was the time everything started to unravel and the investigation began. It didn't take many words to start it: "Can you tell me how I go about reporting childhood sexual abuse, as I am scared other children may be at risk?"

Was this easy to do? It was much easier than I had initially thought it would be. I believe this is because I had the good fortune of being able to say those initial words to somebody who I already felt safe with. If anybody else is looking to report abuse, I would highly recommend that they have a friend or loved one who they feel safe with to be there with them, as support is something that is so very important throughout this process.

Veronica Westby

Making the Actual Report

The day had come when I was to take that first step into reporting the abusers for the historical abuse I had had to endure as a child. As I wrote in my previous article about this, it was not a decision I had made overnight. I had thought long and hard about the impact this would have on the family members that I was about to bring to the forefront. I had equally thought long and hard about what implications it may have on my own children, who were now grown adults living their own independent lives. I had thought about the friends I had and discussed my intentions with them all. I had already, at this stage, contacted a couple of friends who I knew would be able to give some evidence to verify what I was about to disclose, and they were happy to share what they knew. I had contacted two therapists I had seen to let them know that the police might be in touch and that I was willing to give my permission for any records to be disclosed. At that time I was only able to speak to one of the therapists, as I was having difficulty trying to locate the other, but I wasn't going to let that stop me from doing what I knew I had to do to try and prevent other children suffering. I had spoken to a couple of dear friends in the US who I knew were going to be my pillars of strength throughout this. I thought I had covered every base to ensure this next stage of the journey would go as smoothly as it possibly could.

I already knew that this was possibly going to be one of the hardest things I had ever done. Emotionally it would test me to my limits. I won't deny there were times I questioned whether I was doing the right thing or not. However, for every question, the face of a child would appear in my mind's eye. Could I turn my back on that image and just ignore it? No, I couldn't. I had a strong voice in my head that would say to me, "Look at how many times nobody checked on you, can you do the same?" That was to become the voice of strength for me during this stage.

With a strong cup of coffee next to me, a packet of cigarettes close by, and the screen of the survivors support forum up visible on my computer to help me feel close to people who were supporting me, I dialed the number.

I was fortunate in knowing a member of the local police force, as I can only imagine how much harder it would have been to have started this with a complete stranger. So, in a way, by talking to this officer, it was as if I were testing myself to see if I was strong enough to go through with this. I only had to say to her: "I need you to come round, as I need to talk to you about getting advice on how to report child abuse that happened to me as a child."

It did feel as though my life stood still for a bit then. It was probably no more than a few seconds, but not for me, hyper alert, listening to every sound at the other end of that phone, listening to see if I could hear intakes of breath, hesitation, a stuttering of words, anything, just anything to give me a clue as to what her reaction to this was. I know that a part of me was expecting to be brushed away and ignored, just as I had always done as a child.

Instead I got her usual confident and calm voice saying to me, "Ok, I will be round in half an hour." Upon placing the phone receiver down, I sat there feeling stunned for a while. The only way to describe what was going on for me at that moment is to say that time almost felt as though it had been frozen. In reality, it was me that had frozen, as this was the part of me coming forward that had been programmed by the abusers to stay silent. I had finally started the ball rolling on breaking that silence, thus breaking their programming. I do believe, on looking back at that moment, that I had become frozen as this was a new path I was now venturing on. A new path that was totally alien to the very core of my being. I was about to embark into a forest that was totally unknown to me. I had moved into the freeze stage, an area I was not as familiar with as the flight or fright areas that I had grown accustomed to throughout my whole life. From my own training as a therapist, I knew I had to work hard now to move from this stage or I would be unable to proceed any further, and I was on a tight schedule as the officer was due on my doorstep in a very short time.

I knew that in order to break the physical feelings of being frozen, I had to move. I had to give myself the permission to move - so I, as daft as it sounds, told myself I needed to make sure the room was tidy. I am in no way a house-proud person, but I know I hold a huge amount of shame inside if anybody arrives to visit and there isn't some element of tidiness in my home. This shame was actually to be my saving grace, as it gave me the push that I needed to break out of the cycle of being frozen. I know from my past patterns of behavior that if I hadn't broken through this, I would not have even answered the door upon the officer's arrival. So there I was pottering around the room, tidying up a few things, feeling numb. I guess, looking back, I was possibly in a sort of shock state. I had said some very powerful words which were now going to potentially change my whole life.

The doorbell rings... That's when all of a sudden I feel a massive pounding in my chest, almost racing, I can feel my heart trying to leap out of my ribcage. I can hear my blood pulsating in my ears. I look through the peephole to see the officer stood there. I take a deep breath, hoping she can't hear my heart beating like I can, and open the door. She is not on her own, she is with a colleague that I also know. That was not what I had emotionally prepared for, or even thought would happen. Now what was I to do? It made sense in my rational thinking that she would have a colleague with her, as police officers don't work alone, and considering what I was about to disclose to her, it wouldn't have been ethical or legally safe for her to see me on my own. I had two options: I could either say I was not going to take this further or carry on.

I invited them both in and asked them to sit down; I offered them both a hot drink, which to my relief they accepted, as this gave me the few minutes alone in my kitchen to take a deep breath and to regroup my thoughts and feelings. I was able to tell myself that the colleague wasn't a stranger to me as I had met her on many other occasions. It was a tough few moments for me to say the least. Looking back it was almost as though I had been given the option to stop here and now if I chose to. I knew in my heart, though, that I would more than likely have to tell my story to many strangers in the future, so why not use this time to get used to it? It seems almost flippant saying 'get used to it'. In reality, would I ever get used to disclosing the abuse I endured as a child? I didn't know the answer to that, but I did know the reason why I was coming forward now was to try and protect other children, so with that in mind, I walked back through from the kitchen with drinks in hand, ready to continue what I knew I needed to do.

After general chatting about mundane things to do with my area and crime levels etc, I found myself not knowing how to even approach the subject. I had again become frozen inside. I could feel my stomach churning and my heart beating, but it was almost as if the words were stuck in the bottom of my stomach. I couldn't say anything. The police officer looked at me and smiled, she then told me she had spoken to her senior before coming to see me as this was a totally new area, and she had no experience of dealing with historical abuse. I found myself physically relaxing, as I smiled at her and said, 'Well, I have.' My humour, again, was going to carry me through this.

I was able to give her a very brief view of what my concerns were. I told her how I had found that the brother had a website and he had innocent-looking photographs of children as young as seven on his website that he was saying he teaches guitar to. I was able to tell her that, to the best of my knowledge, I knew these guitar lessons to have been taking place in his own bedroom unsupervised and, more recently, in a studio that had been built at the side of his home. Fortunately at this time I didn't have to go into details of the abuse I had endured at his hands, but just enough information to clarify that I felt I had been sexually abused by him when I was younger. I also was able to disclose that the father also lived in this house too and he, too, had sexually abused me at the young age of three.

With that information imparted, I knew that I had started the ball rolling. I knew that this would now go onto official records. At this stage I didn't need to give any further information. I had made the allegations. I also showed the website to the officer so that she could verify that she, too, had seen the images of the children, albeit innocent images of them holding guitars.

The officer then informed me that the next stage was that she would need to go back to the station and make a report of what I had shared with her to the police officers in charge of the Child Protection Team. They would then be in contact with me to take down more details. I don't think I was really expecting this, I think I felt that I would only have to tell one person and then it could all go from there, so that was a bit of a shock to me. It did make sense though, as obviously they were going to need to know the history in more depth.

After the officer left my home, I felt as though I was on a bit of a rollercoaster ride. Part of me felt guilty for breaking the family secret, part of me felt relieved that I was actually doing something to make sure these other children were safe. I also found myself feeling very scared, of what I really don't know, maybe it was stemming from the small child in me who had for so many years been silenced, finally somebody had actually heard her and was going to investigate what I had said.

I was alone in my home, which looking back was a big mistake. I found the next few hours quite harrowing; I had opened up 'Pandora's box' on my emotions of guilt and fear. I had to sit with those emotions on my own. I found I camped out on the Survivors' Forum just so I could feel close to people who understood how I was feeling. I didn't really have anybody I could ask to just come and sit with me. What I think would have been much better and an even more productive distraction would have been to have gone out, even if it had just been for a coffee at the local coffee shop. In hindsight and I would recommend this to anyone who makes the decision to report historical abuse - make sure you have somebody with you who you trust. Don't be alone, and make sure you have a support network so that if one person isn't available, then you can call on someone else.

Veronica Westby

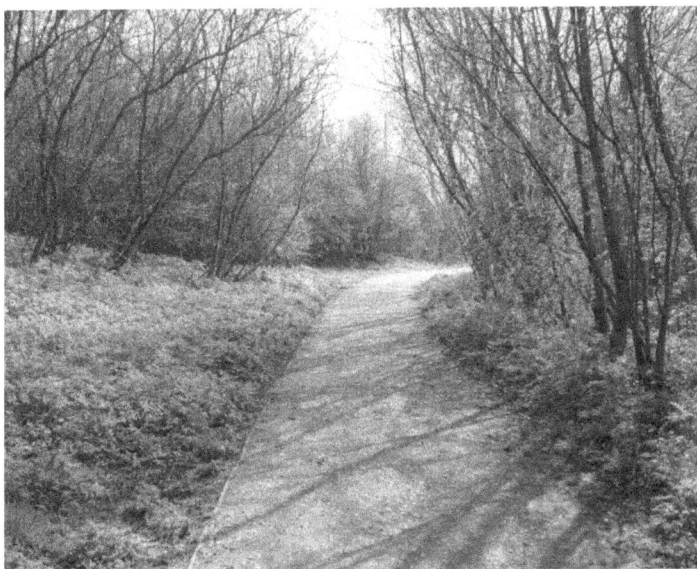

'No one finds life worth living; he must make it worth
living.'

Author unknown

Choices

I didn't choose to be born to a young catholic girl whose
parents wouldn't support her.
I didn't choose to be adopted through the Catholic Church.
I didn't choose my adoptive parents.
I didn't choose to be locked in the toilet and tied sat on the
toilet.
I didn't choose to be sexually abused by my adoptive father
at the aged of two.
I didn't choose to be beaten with sticks, canes, wooden
spoons, belts and riding whips.
I didn't choose to be taken to ritualistic ceremonies in Africa.
I didn't choose to be locked in the larder.
I didn't choose to be locked in the shed.
I didn't choose to be locked in the bedroom.
I didn't choose to be locked in the caravan.
I didn't choose to be called 'ape'.
I didn't choose to be sexually abused by those two old men.
I didn't choose for my brother to sexually abuse me.
I didn't choose for the neighbour to drag me round by my
hair and beat me until near unconsciousness for mother.
I didn't choose to be so thirsty I would drink out of the toilet
or dog's bowl.
I didn't choose to have to eat my own faeces.
I didn't choose to have to pee in a bucket.
I didn't choose not to be able to have clothes.
I didn't choose to be so cold I would have chilblains on my
hands and feet.
I didn't choose to be bullied at school.
I didn't choose not to be loved.
I didn't choose to not be heard.
I didn't choose to be ignored.
I didn't choose many things as a child.
The one choice I never had which I do now is
The choice of freedom.

Veronica Westby

A Prayer and a Revelation

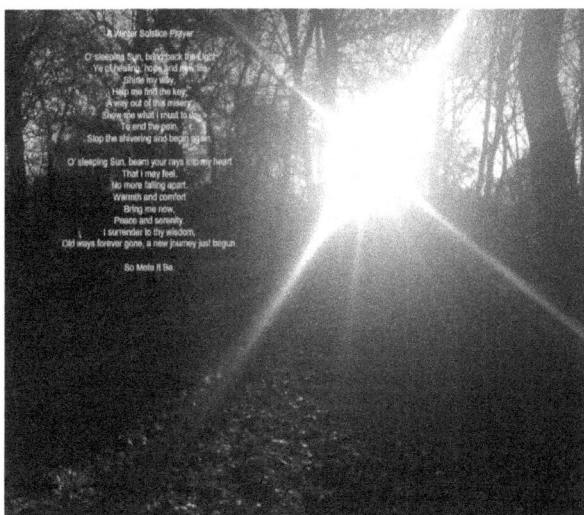

I ˈsent out a message to the spirit world on 22nd December 2005 that I didn't want to live like this anymore: putting on an act, saying the 'right' things, struggling to appear composed while fighting against inner trembling, nausea, panic attacks and phobias. I was 40 years old, exhausted and weary from years of living in a state of high alert; a half personality, half a brain, half a spirit, half a soul. I felt fake and a hypocrite. No one had a clue as to what I was going through, and no one cared. I loathed the fact that I couldn't go out anywhere without a stash of herbal sedatives and a disguised bottle of brandy. I hated my body and I hated myself.

On that longest, darkest night of the year, I joined a Winter Solstice celebration in South London on the invitation of two friends. After all the singing and circle dancing and saying our farewells to the past year, we lit candles and placed them around the Yule log to send out light and positive energy to cast away problems. The ceremony and the gentle nature of the people soothed my tension and replaced inner turmoil with peace. In that quiet, still space I whispered my own prayer for a new beginning, for a new light to shine in my world and cast away my problems, confusion and suffering.

Later that evening, I logged onto my laptop to surf the web in search of finding out the meaning of a friend's bi-polar medical condition. I found myself scrolling down a page about Post-Traumatic Stress Disorder (PTSD) in rape survivors and to my surprise discovered that I was reading about myself. I couldn't take my eyes off the screen. Never before had anyone articulated how I felt with such insight, clarity and understanding.

It hadn't even occurred to me that I might have a 'disorder' or health condition with recognisable symptoms. I had never considered myself as ill, just battling on in life, trying to function normally while my body did weird things. It felt as if my prayers had been answered. A bright light had illuminated a dark and forgotten corner of my world. I had been heard... All I had to do now was find the right person to set me on the road to recovery.

A Winter Solstice Prayer

O' sleeping Sun, bring back the Light
Ye of healing, hope and new life
Shine my way,
Help me find the key,
A way out of this misery.
Show me what I must to do
To end the pain,
Stop the shivering and begin again.

O' sleeping Sun, beam your rays into my
heart
That I may feel,
No more falling apart.
Warmth and comfort
Bring me now,
Peace and serenity.
I surrender to thy wisdom,
Old ways forever gone, a new journey just
begun.

So Mote It Be.

Based on journal extracts, December 2005

By Angelite

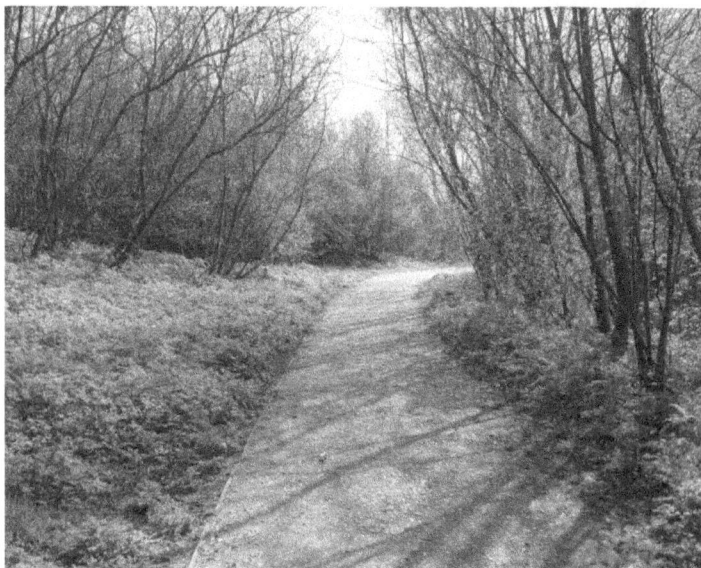

"I will be me. I won't be second best for anyone."

Wendy Johnson

Healing is...

Hearing the deep call from within,
the soul calling you Home.

Seeing the walls that enclose you, and
making a promise to yourself to find the way out.
Starting the search for answers.
Accepting that everyone's path is going to be different.
There is no 'right way' or 'wrong way', only little steps.

Allowing your heart to guide you.
Trusting that what is right for you will appear at the right
time.
Keeping faith that things will get better.
Unravelling the myths & fairy tales that defined you
Discovering who you really are.
Learning to love yourself.
Seeing rainbows when it's raining.
Allowing emotions to surface without fear or judgement.
You've been through a lot. It's normal.
Welcoming tears when they come.
They are releasing pain and old hurts.
Trusting and honouring your instincts.
They will guide and protect you.
Forgiving yourself for all that happened.
You did the best you could at the time...
That was how you survived.

Angelite

I SURVIVE

Is this the way we were made?

So much pain we had to endure

Until someone believed our stories

Revival of our spirits began

Venturing into a whole new world

Interpreting our living hells

Vindicating ourselves from blame and shame

Each of us learning to strive for our freedom.

Veronica Westby

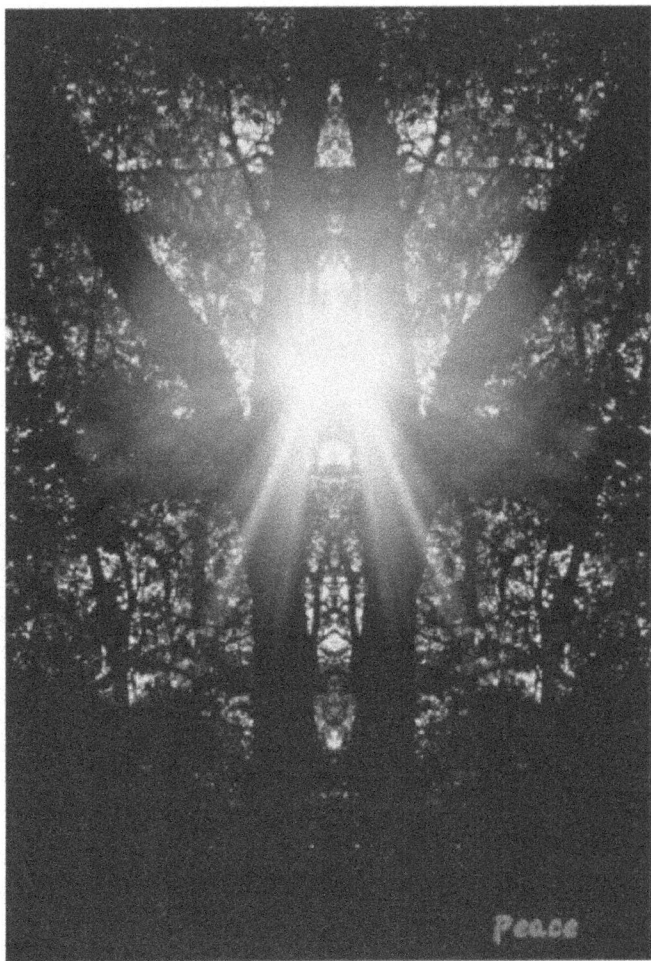

'Peace'

Photograph by Denise Claxton

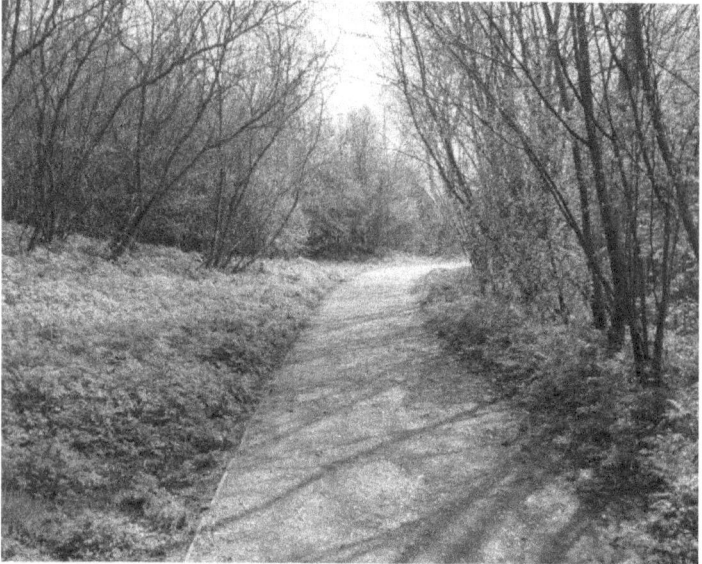

"If you're not being treated with love and respect, check your price tag. Perhaps you've marked yourself down. It's YOU who tell people what you're worth by what you accept. Get off the clearance rack and get behind the glass where they keep the valuables! Bottom Line: Value yourself more! If you don't then no one will. I'm priceless! Are you?"

Author unknown

Plea to Hospital Staff

Please just don't dismiss me
'Cause I've turned up here again
Overdosed and cut myself
I really need some help

Please just don't condemn me
'Cause I don't reflect the norm
Every time I cut myself
The feelings begin to dawn

Please don't misunderstand me
When I walk back through your door
I really don't want to be here
But don't you slam that door

Please don't you try and judge me
By behaviour that you see
Just try and understand me
And look beyond my scars to me

Please look beyond the scars and cuts
And see there's me inside
Trying hard to make it through
And rebuild all of my pride

So please just don't chastise me
It really doesn't help
Neither will it stop me
When all you do is shout

Please remember I'm an adult
Although I feel just like a child
But treat me like a baby
And I'll behave just like a child

So please just don't dismiss me
When I return yet again
And please just try and help me
So I can function once again.

Lynn Alston

The Lottery We Don't Want To Play

Today I spoke to an adult survivor in her 40s, and she said she was ready to get some help for the past that was weighing her down so badly. What a wonderful and brave decision she has made... How does society honour and support her decision to get help for something which was not within her control? Where is the specialist help? I was one of the lucky ones, after a few not-so-great counsellors I had a fantastic person who helped me more than ever. Sadly, now it has become even more of a lottery, in terms of what help you get and for how long. This really needs looking at from a government level. Often people seem to forget that these children grow up and have to live with this legacy - surely as a society we should be doing all we can to help them restore their lives? Instead, the perpetrators seem all too often to get more help than the victims. It is so distorted - time for change!

Kate Swift

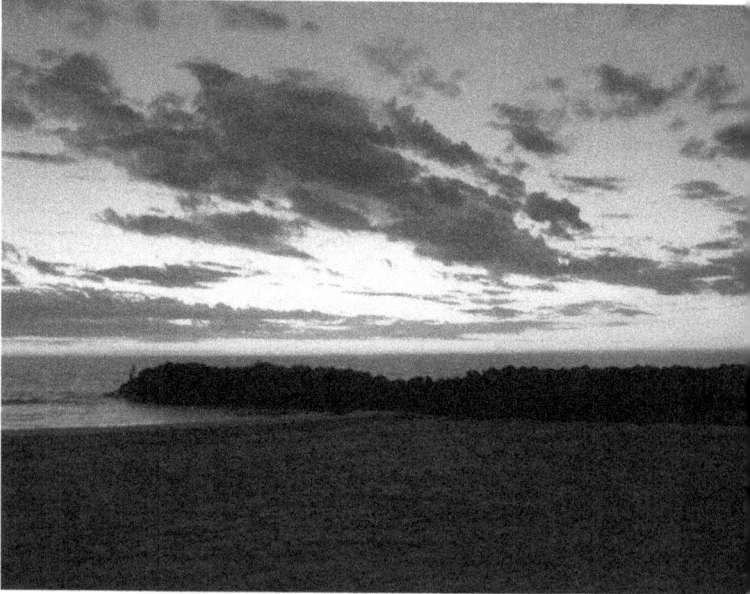

"With each sunset comes the dawn of a new day, and all the hopes and dreams that it contains."

Words and photograph by Ray Redner

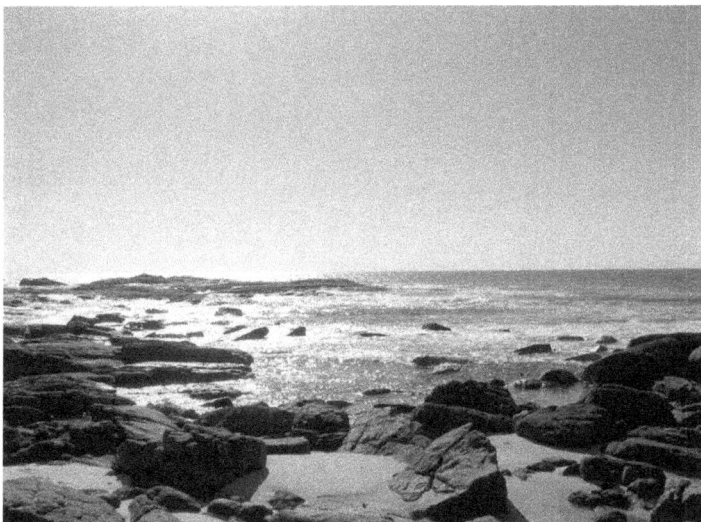

"Sometimes recovery can be smooth seas and picturesque scenes, but other times it can be raging waters breaking upon the rocks. Both sorts of seasons are necessary to learn how to grow stronger and endure - to be more than survivors, but to become conquerors."

Words and photograph by Ray Redner

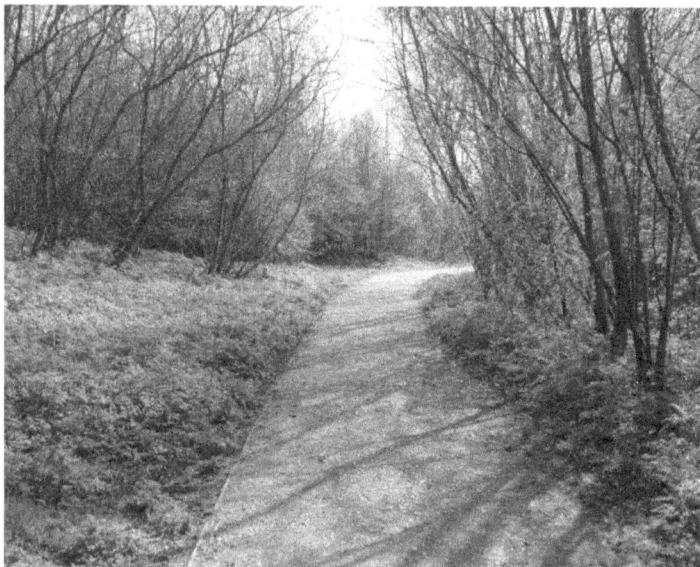

"I'm somebody and I DO matter."

Michelle Shelley Taylor

Silence is not golden

Silence is brutal. Silence is cruel. Silence is binding.

Silence is so powerful that after the first time my uncle raped me, I began to stutter so badly that it was nearly impossible to understand anything I said. I was literally bound and gagged by my own mouth. The horror and confusion and trauma were trapped inside, wrapped up in a tight bandage of silence, eradicating any possibility of speaking.

Truth was trapped by my silence, and I have lived with the repercussions of that my entire life, the way that a stone dropped into a pond creates innumerable ripples spreading out to the edges of the bank. All the years that truth was screaming, clawing, burning, and flailing away inside to be given life and freedom, silence held it captive. I did not know how destructive silence would be, how tenaciously I held onto the belief that relinquishing silence would be the catalyst for the implosion of my world.

I have found my voice.

I have chosen sound over silence, truth over deception, and light over darkness. The consequences of my choice have been great, but I will never again be a captive to silence. I will share my truth, and speak it when it would otherwise be quieted.

I am an advocate for truth, and a destroyer of Silence.

Silence is not golden.

Jess Reece
http://www.jlreece.blog.com/

Christmas was hard. Or rather, the days leading up to Christmas were hard. I couldn't help but be acutely aware of how different this year is compared to previous years - of how utterly broken all connections to my mother are now. It makes me sad. But also … lighter … somehow.
The day after Christmas I felt as though a weight had disappeared from my shoulders. The ghost of her brutal betrayal feels far away now - not gone completely, but no longer bending me to the ground in emotional submission. A lot of my anger is gone now as well. I'm sure some of that is there, too, but it doesn't feel like toxic sludge oozing through me anymore.

I just don't want to give up any more of myself to her.

In order to do that, I have to clear out this emotional pollution, replacing it with clean, clear peace and happiness. Next year is for *me*. It will get the real me, the shining, amazing *me* that has been hidden under years of tarnish. I have to unearth the side of me that shows my true potential - give freedom to the creativity inside demanding to see the light of day. It's like when you finally get to take off that heavy winter coat because spring is here!

This coming year holds enormous potential - so much promise, just waiting for me to tap into it. One of my favourite sayings is by Ralph Waldo Emerson: "The creation of a thousand forests is in one acorn." The tiniest seed (of anything really) has the inherent potential to grow into great things. And not just one thing, but from that potential sprouts a thousand other things. That potential is there, just waiting for the right set of circumstances to encourage it to grow, to change, to *become*.

I am surrounded by love and light right now, and I feel that it is time for me to embrace my potential, to begin fulfilling my purpose. I have the healthy nourishment I need to grow, and have removed the toxic factors that were holding me back before. I am truly free to find *me*.

Jess Reece
http://www.jlreece.blog.com/

My Victory

You chose your weapons
leaving me no shield
no protection, no safety
a prisoner in your lair

It was your fancy and your delight
to watch me cower and tremble
not able to fight

You waged war and brutality
against me, a small child
bruised, battered, bloodied
you chanted your victory shout

Believing you had won the battle
over time you fell
death, insanity, madness, overtook you
and your frame returned to dust

A small wounded child grew
amongst the thorns
she learned along the path from teachers
wise and true

They taught her to learn to love herself
taught her to love others
they planted a spark of light within
that grew as time moved on

Today that small girl is grown,
and stands tall
She faced her demons, faced her death
and learned to love and live.

Laurie Ann Smith, 2012

http://www.lulu.com/spotlight/LaurieAnnSmith

http://www.blogtalkradio.com/laurie-smith

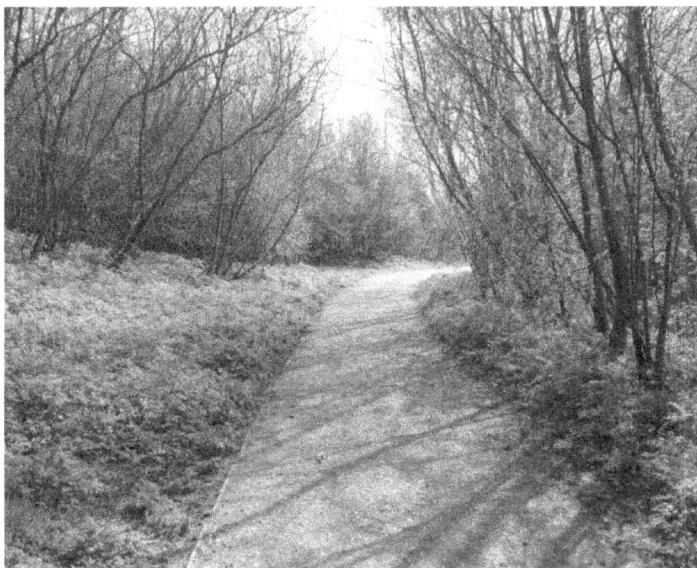

"One day I will shine and I will walk on untouched snow
and be at peace within myself."

Wendy Johnson

Brush Away Your Tears

Brush away the tears from your eyes, my child
The world don't want to see you cry
Brush away the tears from your eyes, my child
The world don't want to hear you cry

And though it's not right you've got to carry on with your
life – please try
The world don't understand, sticks its head in the sand -
and hides
I wish I could take your hand, try to help you understand
my child
You've got to carry on; your story must be told –
sometime

Brush away the tears from your eyes, my child
The world don't want to see you cry
Brush away the tears from your eyes, my child
The world don't want to hear you cry

When you're standing all alone, reach inside to carry on
- dear child
Find the ways to be strong, though they may break you
down inside
Your spirit is still alive so look around and you'll find
A friend who'll hold your hand, will try their best to
understand your life
So till then please carry on, find the ways to be strong
my child

Brush away the tears from your eyes, my child
The world don't want to see you cry
Brush away the tears from your eyes, my child
The world don't want to hear you cry

Brush away your tears
Hide all of your fears
Hide all of your pain
Hide all of your shame
The world don't want to know
The world don't want to know

Someday the world will understand
And then they'll hold out their hand
'Til then you must be strong
And find the way to carry on
Brush away your tears
Brush away your tears

Song by Michael C. Skinner
www.mskinnermusic.com
www.survivingspirit.com

About *Brush Away Your Tears*

"Brush away the tears from your eyes my child, the world don't want to see you cry," are the opening lines to this song, which I wrote in October 2005. These words pretty much summed up what I was feeling at the time – sad and disillusioned after many years of advocacy in raising awareness on the issues and concerns of child abuse.

Music has always been a powerful way to express my feelings whether as a drummer, singer, songwriter and/or guitarist. I found the writing of this song helped to capture and convey what I was feeling at that time in my life. I had been involved in public speaking and performing songs addressing child abuse since 1993 and once again I was being asked to present at the *Children in Slavery - The 21st Century Summit* conference. This powerful event was addressing the plight of those being victimized in the trafficking trade – I was asked to present as a childhood survivor of trafficking.

I was honored to participate in this important event being co-sponsored by the United Nations, The United States State Department and Georgetown University – but there was a part of me that wondered whether this would be just one experience of sharing and my words, and the words of others would fall upon deaf ears. Thus, the song was written to help express my feelings and thoughts that shared my frustration of how so many look the other way when it comes to child abuse and yet the song would offer hope to those impacted by their respective abuse.

Michael C. Skinner

www.mskinnermusic.com

www.survivingspirit.com

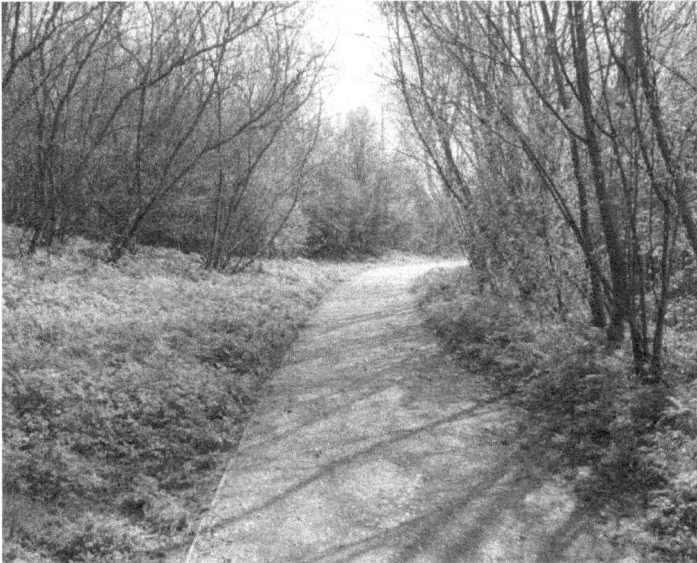

"I am so proud of me... been there before, not going there again!"

Michelle Shelley Taylor

Our healing wishes
for all
survivors

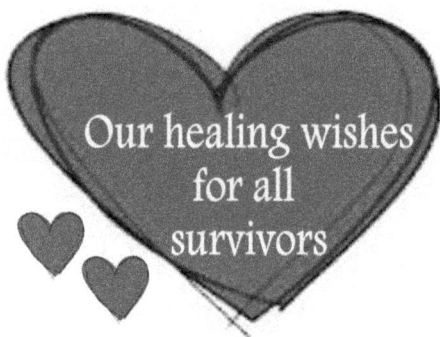

My healing wish for all survivors is... For someone to look you in the eye and tell you the truth: that what happened to you was NOT your fault. For strength and endurance to face each day, particularly those days when all you want to do is curl up and hide from the whole world. To know that things can and do get better... to know that you deserve to be safe & happy... to know that you deserve to live the life of your dreams and to have the courage to chase them. *Kate Swift*

My healing wish for all survivors is... Face the fear head on. There's no looking back, be true to you in your fight to heal everyone else can wait. *Wendy Johnson*

My healing wish for all survivors is... That they manage to find all the precious pieces of their shattered selves and become whole. *Meryl Aves*

My healing wish for all survivors is... to stop the prejudice in society. *Deb*

My healing wish for all survivors is... to never give up, to always have friends and groups like R.S.O.S.A to help with the healing process, to be honest with yourselves and with others and to be accepted for who you are. *Sheila Cooper*

My healing wish for all survivors is... that we all find the strength to move forward without the fear of the future. *Jo Descoteaux*

My healing wish for all survivors is... to accept help and support to get us through the hard time we have as we make our journey. *Angela Steer*

My healing wish for all survivors is... that all of us survivors eventually find the peace and strength to move on with our lives, and we can live out or hopes and dreams as we so very much deserve. *Katrina Pacey*

My healing wish for all survivors is... that we could all get better one day and for people to understand what goes on in someone's head when they commit suicide. *Gemma Merrick*

My healing wish for all survivors is... to keep strong and to have a happy life. *Wendy Lawson*

My healing wish for all survivors is... for each of us to be able to stand tall, look the world in the eye and say, "Look at me. I have been through the flames of hell, yet look at how strong I have become despite those who wished to silence me and make me weak." *Pete Burton*

My healing wish for all survivors is... that my training goes well to become a police officer so I can help survivors. *Jessa*

My healing wish for all survivors is... to see true recovery come to fruition so that feelings of peace surround them, and as confidence grows they can go on to help others. *Nicky Palmer*

My healing wish for all survivors is... that they can learn to love themselves and that they can reclaim and live their lives to the fullest with all of the love, joy and peace that they deserve. Loving yourself is the foundation of all real healing. *Patricia Singleton*

Growing Stronger, Growing Free

My healing wish for all survivors is... that we hold our heads high and realise it was not then nor will it ever be our fault and we CAN move forward with love and support from one another and those who truly love us. *Victoria Barto*

My healing wish for all survivors is... that they can be accepted and loved unconditionally and to be able to believe in that acceptance and love. *Lindsay Greenwood*

My healing wish for all survivors is... one that has already been mentioned but worth mentioning again: to never, ever give up - things do get better even when you think they won't; to stand tall and be proud of who you are always; and to know you are cherished by those who really do care for you, that you are indeed special. *Mary Gypsy*

My healing wish for all survivors is... that you believe that you are WORTHY of love, peace, and happiness... because you are. *Jess Reece*

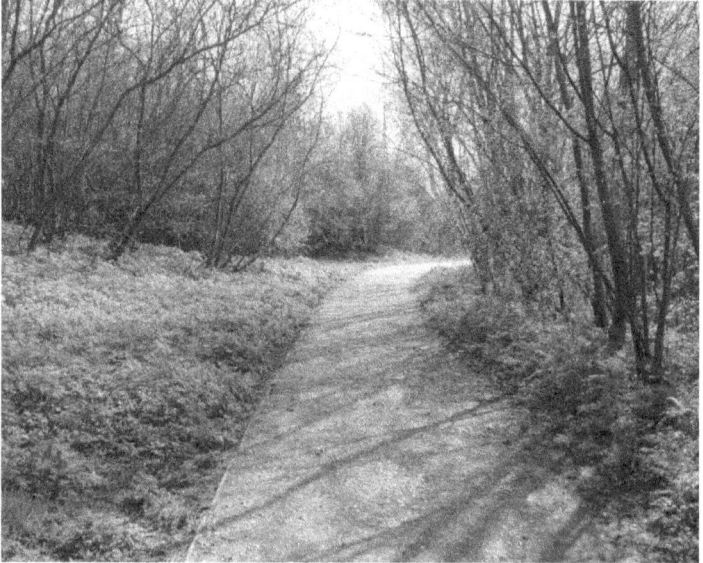

"Think highly of yourself, for the world takes you at your own estimate."

Author unknown

Victim or Survivor?

Hidden secrets of which nobody knows,
Dirty little lies & painful violent blows,
My tears of pain & the silent screams,
It's your cruel actions that haunt my dreams.

For the pain to stop I begged & pleaded,
My yells of pain that no-one ever heeded,
You hurt me more & held me still,
You did such awful things against my will.

As a child my spirit was bruised & broken,
Of what you had done I'd never spoken,
Years have passed since those dreadful days,
Yet bruised & broken I remain in so many ways.

Not quite alive nor yet totally dead,
What you have done has left deep scars within my
head,
In my mind & in my soul,
What you did has left a gaping hole.

All that hurt that you have caused to me,
Has left me with demons that haunt & torment me,
You stole my innocence & hurt me so,
I trusted you completely but you have left me feeling so
hollow.

In both my mind & my heart,
Your sick actions tore me apart,
I was just a child so innocent & meek,
Yet you left me feeling so afraid & weak.

Now however I know what you did was so wrong,
Although the pain is still there I'm trying to fight & be
strong,
What you have done to me will not keep me broken,
I will stand tall from my nightmares once I have woken.

I will grow each day & do my best I shall but try,
I will overcome this pain & not let my spirit die,
Although what you did to me hurts me still,
I will never give up nor surrender my free will.

Although it has taken me a while to get where I am,
I am fighting this fight because win it I know that I can,
I am no longer the weak child that you once knew today
I am a strong fighter,
I know without a shadow of a doubt that I am a survivor

Tori Hollinshead

Who am I, I do not know,
Am I a friend or am I a foe?
Am I kind or am I cruel?
Am I serious or do I act the fool?
I am a survivor of abuse or at least I think I am,
I sometimes feel my life has been a complete sham,
Abuse brings with it many faults,
Self harm, suicide, self blame, it's a scary jaunt,
I am me, just me, do you think you know me?
Do you see through my mask of deceit?
Do you see my deepest, darkest fears?
Do you see through the fake smile to my inner tears?
Do you understand me, do you see the real me,
The one that hides from my reality,
I am the one that fought for justice & won,
I am the one who should be saying my life has now
begun,
I should be able to move on from this should I not?
I feel lost in the world of forget-me-nots,
I am but one small voice of thousands,
I was heard, believed but yet I feel lousy,
My life for all that it has been,
Has yet to begin, has yet to be truly seen.

Tori Hollinshead

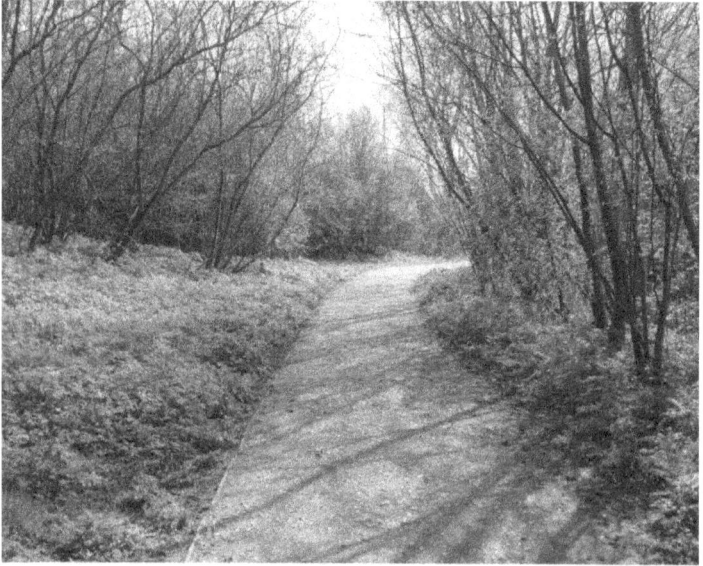

"Don't forget to look back just long enough to see how far forward you have come."

Kate Swift

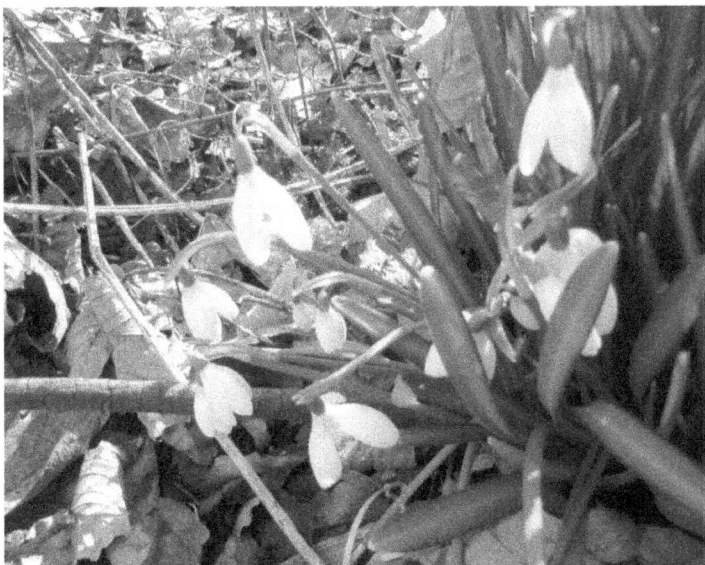

Dark winter holds life in iron fist
Ground cold, hard as steel
Impenetrable
But wait
Battling through this impossible challenge
A Snowdrop
Delicate and beautiful
Victorious against the cold hard ground
A beacon to warm the heart
A harbinger of Hope and better things.

Photograph and poem by Pete Burton

I hate my body and I hate my soul,
I hate my life and I have no goals.
I hate the winter, but I love the spring,
I like the new year, when positive things begin.
I hate my scars but I love the stars.
I don't like rhyming my every word, but I do like
sounding a bit absurd.
I have a mum but I don't have a dad, I have a brother
who is a bit mad. I am a sister and I am a daughter, but
if I was a sheep I'd rather be slung to slaughter.
I'd run to where ever my feet could take me, somewhere
where people wouldn't hate me.
I love my recovery, every step of the way, I have been in
darkness, and without help I wouldn't be here today.
My point in life is what I desire; my love for poetry gets
me admirers.
Life is simple, when you have your goals, but because
of depression I am stuck on hold.
Pause the memories, and stop the hate, before you turn
around and it's too late.
We are survivors, and survivors we stand strong, we
don't fight or argue, we all get along.
Recovery is magical, every step of the way, so don't be
afraid to admit it, don't be so ashamed.
I love you all, as you are my family, despite all the
obstacles we can all still believe!

Gemma Merrick

Life

I am so lucky, come look at me
See what I have seen, what I've achieved
Come listen for a while and listen real good
Will tell you how it started, but the start was not
good

Once upon a time a long while ago
There once lived a very scared little girl
Bubbly and bright filled with delight
Taken from her pure innocent light

But she grew up and grew very strong
Took on the world and all that belong
Fighting back and getting herself strong
Learning to live with whatever was to become
She gave it her all she tried all she could,
But finally gave the will to fight

Now it's new and time to get on
She's now got friends who helped her grow back
being strong
Gave her confidence with grace and a smile
Told her what she needed to go that extra mile
Now she's working and growing strong each day
They see her smile they see her laugh
Because now she's on the right path

So it's not all sad, it's a learning curve
Be yourself and never controlled
Not by yourself not by your love
Be happy, be smiley, be who you want to be
'Cause I will tell you something now
I'm finally back being me.

Wendy Lawson

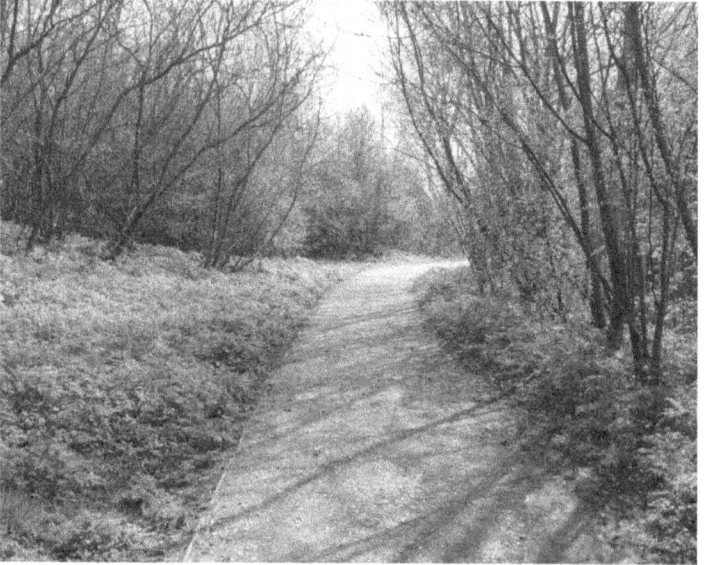

"Put your abuser where they belong and put yourself on the healing road. They do not deserve to steal another minute of your life... take back your power and walk."

Anon

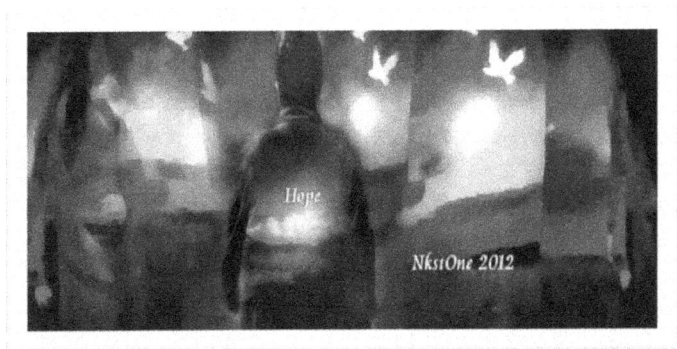

By Nikki Stone

My name is Kenneth Doyle, author of *Mummy from Hell*. For the first sixteen years of my life, my brother Patrick and I were abused by our own mother in Ireland. Our abuse was in the form of starvation, daily beatings and all forms of torture our mother could inflict upon us. I got out of my home at age sixteen and made my own way through life. I never returned home and never had any desire to return.

Once I was away from home I took up drinking. I found that when I was drunk I could numb my past. I had no idea that there was anything wrong with me. But I was remembering my past. I was waking up in the middle of the night crying. I would be dreaming of my abuse. During the day I always flash back to my abuse. I thought this was normal. I did find that once I was drunk I would not flash back to the abuse. When I awoke during the night I would have a beer. I did my best to stay drunk. Drink took over my life.

About eleven years ago I received hundreds of pages of medical files from Ireland. To my shock and horror I read from my files where all of those around me knew that we were being abused from when we were only toddlers. I was angry. I decided to go and talk to someone about my drinking problem. I noticed that after I got the files I was drinking a little more and I was getting very sad while drunk. When I told my therapist about my abuse she was shocked and told me the reason I was drinking was that I was suffering from post traumatic stress disorder (PTSD). She explained what PTSD is and how it has a lasting effect on victims of abuse. I was told that in order to get help I would have to quit the drink. This is not what I wanted to hear, but it was up to me.

Seven years ago I made a big step. I gave up alcohol and have no desire to return to it. I am in counselling and attend twice a month. I am taking a couple of medications for PTSD .Through counselling I have found that my abuse is no longer a secret. I was always under the impression that no one knew. During my counselling sessions I was given what was like homework. I was asked to write down what my fears were. And what I was flashing back to. Well, over three years of home work I had enough to fill a book. And that is what I did. I decided to write a book to let everyone see what it is like to be an unwanted child. I got together with my brother Patrick and we put our book together .

Our book has done so much for victims that I am thrilled. We have victims contacting us telling us how they too have suffered and how our book has allowed them to come forward with their abuse. We have been contacted by kids who have asked us for help. I am thrilled that I have turned around. I blamed myself for my abuse. I used alcohol as a form of medication. I no longer need the alcohol crutch. I am now helping others who are suffering or have suffered themselves.

Ken Doyle

Tenderness

Advice

Love

Kindness

A person who will listen and not condemn
Someone on whom you can depend;
They will not run when bad times are here
Instead they will be there to lend an ear.

Grant Tribemil

My mind a stormy sea
Crashing back and forth,

No peace.

Mental whirlwind
Making me dizzy,

No peace.

My mind a tornado
Destroying and unsettling,

No peace.

Seek release.
There is no peace;
I am the sky before sunrise
Waiting for the light,
Illuminate the darkness,

Understand direction,
Somehow
PEACE AT LAST!

Grant Tribemil

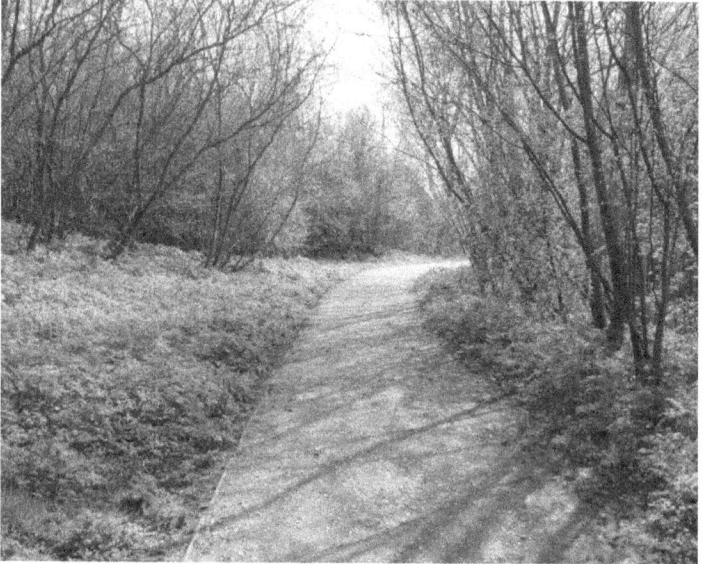

"Wounded people are dangerous; they know they can survive."

Author unknown

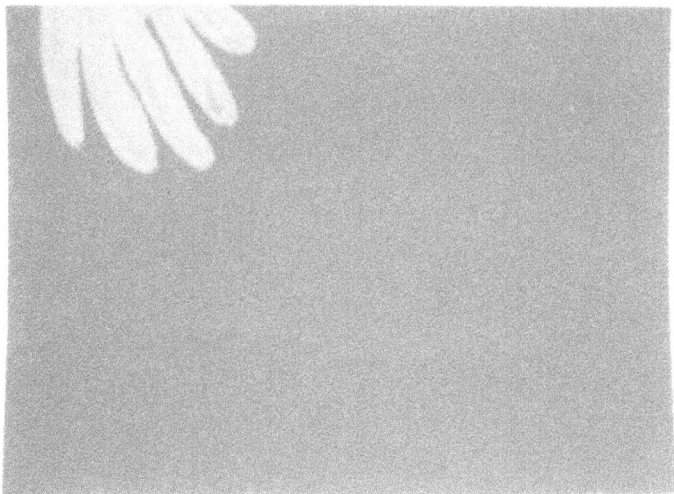

'Take the Help'

Nicky Palmer

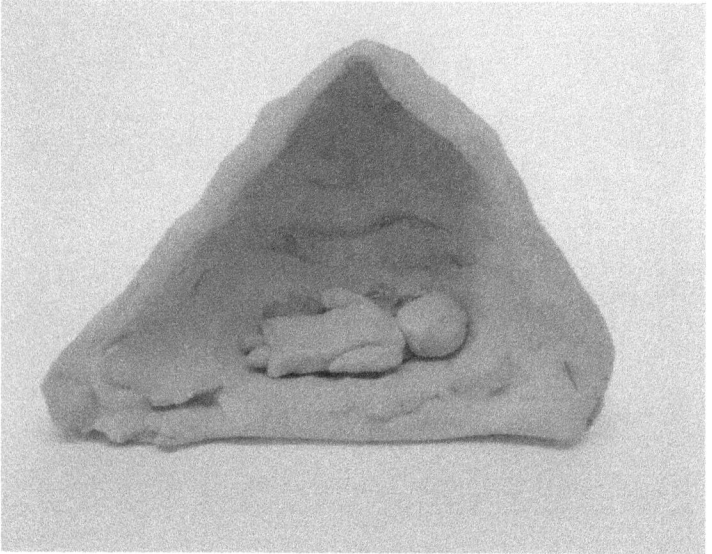

'Perfect'

Nicky Palmer

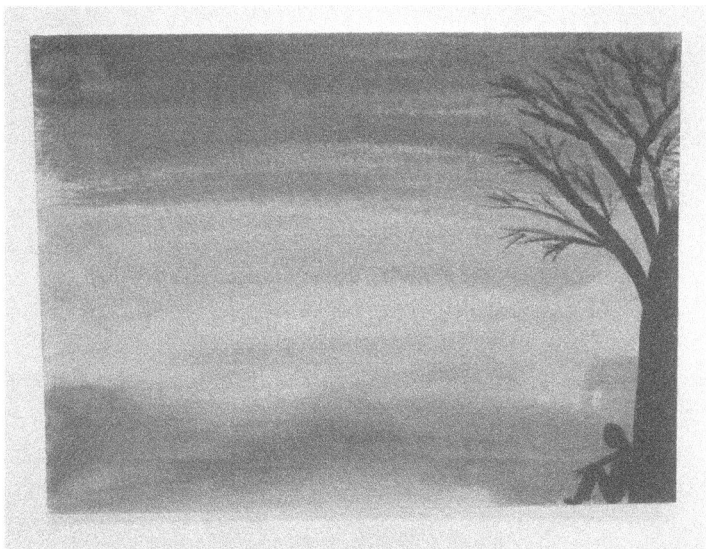

'Hoping'

Nicky Palmer

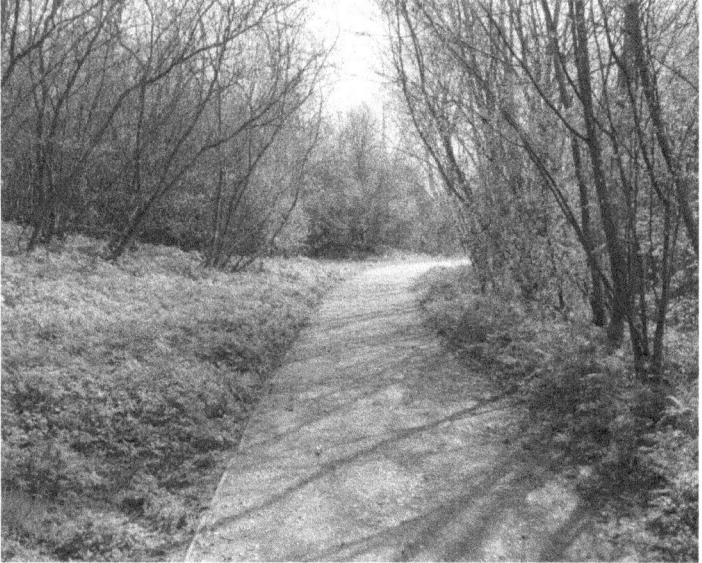

"We, here, are soldiers on the front line of the battle against our shared inner demons. However, whilst we are firing our guns and throwing our grenades, let us not forget to turn back to those still in training, hold their hand and set a good example of how to conquer!"

Nicky Palmer

A Timely Reminder

People who have helped me and seen me grow have told me many times how much I've changed and moved forward for the better. Although I don't see it as much as they do, I think we sometimes need someone to say, "Look how far you have come, don't look back." I know it has been a massive help to me in hard times.

Sheila Cooper

We find SOLACE in…

Our children
Hiding under the duvet
The gym
Running outdoors
A hug
Zumba
Being at the beach
Crafting
Sat quietly in a church
Listening to the sea
Photography
Losing yourself in a 'TV' programme
Being still
Feeling the sun on my face
The freedom to live my own life
Reflecting on progress
Painting and drawing
Music
People watching
Pets
Writing
A bubble bath
Walking in the rain
Watching the snow fall
Scrapbooking
My faith
Chocolate
Helping others
Watching dance
A good book
Long walks in nature
The people who really care about me
Cuddling up to my cat
My daughter's laughter

By Members of R.S.O.S.A

FOOD FOR THE SOUL

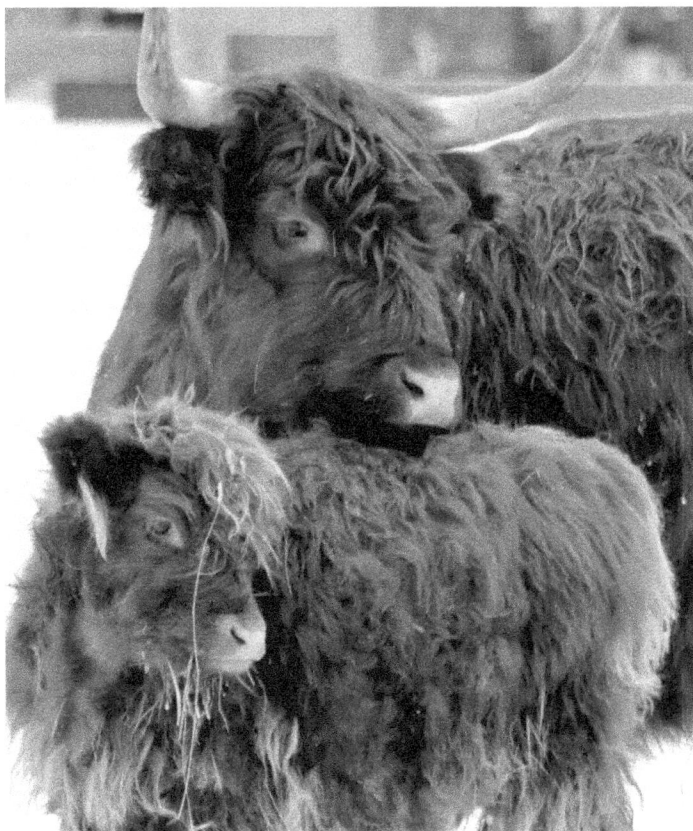

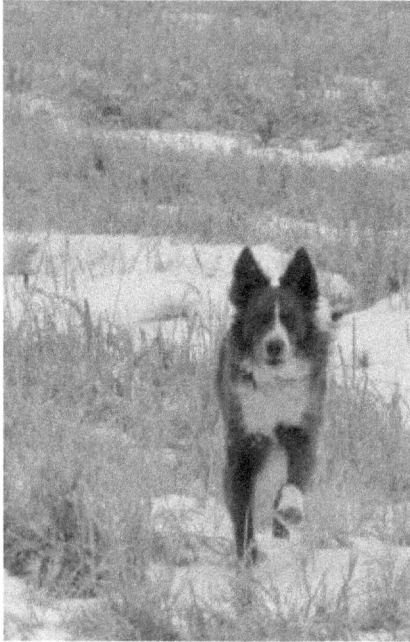

Photography by Shanyn Silinski

FOOD FOR THE SOUL

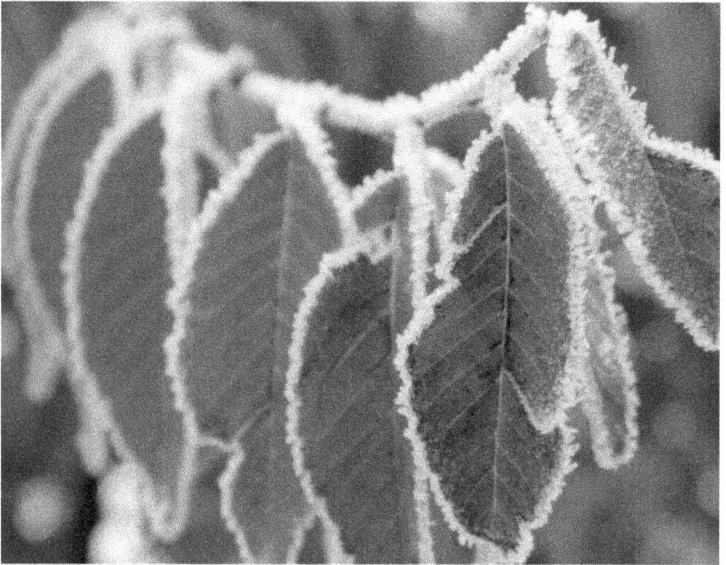

Photography by Shanyn Silinski

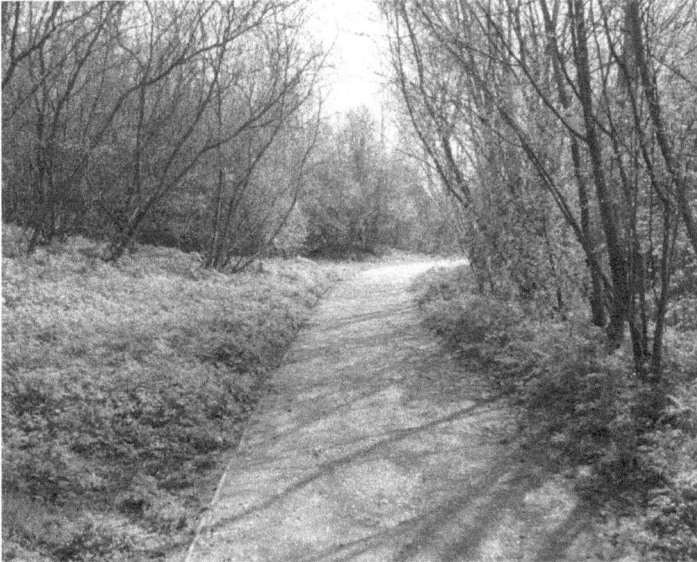

'If you look for the positive things in life, you will find them.'

Author unknown

What being a survivor means to me:

It means having the courage to face the demons of my past and KNOW that I will make it through.

It means knowing that I am free to speak about my abuse because it happened to ME.

It means knowing that my soul really didn't die all those years ago like I thought it did.

It means that I can make it another day and on those days when I feel beaten down... well, that's okay too.

It means knowing deep in my heart that I'm not the only one who has gone through the pain of sexual abuse.

It means being able to reach out and embrace the child that no one seemed to notice.

It means reconnecting me with myself and establishing new relationships on MY terms... not someone else's.

It means feeling love in a safe way and truly understanding what it means and how good it feels to give and receive in a healthy way.

I am nowhere near the end of my journey, but I'm farther than I was before.

I know that I can ask for help when I need it and that it's okay. I won't be judged or told that I'm wrong for feeling the way I do.

I try not to allow people to silence me anymore. It's MY story and MY body and I can choose who I share them with.

I will never be the whole person I was before it happened but I can put the pieces that I have back together again and make a new whole.

It's a new lease on life once in recovery. Growth spurts and new relationships and even new ways of relating to people are what make the pain of the journey worthwhile.

It makes the pain more tolerable when you have somebody by your side who believes in you and will listen to your story without judgement or criticism.

Recovery… it is painful and hard at times, but worth it in the end.

Sarah Walker

How I am healing

The more I speak about it

The freer I feel I am

Even though it hurts extremely much

Working my way free through therapy

It is worth it in the long run.

Speaking the truth sets you free

Even though it is extremely tough.

It's like you're breaking in a thousand pieces,

But the more I speak the more I

Put the pieces back together again

And become the whole me.

It will take the time it needs to take to get there,

Patience and believing it will happen

Brings me forward to heal.

I am growing stronger and growing free.

Janne Helen Tommervåg

Dear Child Within

Your salted droplets keep falling like rain,
while I become weary from feeling your pain.
I'm sorry this evil was laid upon you,
It is over, I'm grown, what more can I do?

You hide, yet you scream "why must it be me?"
I've tasted, I've felt, I've seen what you see.

The pain! It is intense, yet it seems to increase.
Will knowing I love you help make it all cease?

I must be what he couldn't be.
A sibling to guide you, your innocence, set free.

Hush! Don't cry. I know you are sad.
Together we'll make it, life is not all that bad.

I will guard and protect, I'm the adult here outside.
You, the frightened child within, please! don't hide.

Angela Steer

I Am Lucky

I am lucky...
I can feel pain
I can feel love, joy and sadness.

I am lucky...
I have a husband,
Someone who respects me,
Someone who loves me,
Someone who holds me while I weep
and while I rage.

I am lucky...
I have three beautiful children,
Children who respect me,
Children who love me,
Children I can hold and comfort while they weep...
but they do not rage...for that, I am lucky.

I am lucky...
I can smile,
I can laugh,
And I can touch my children with tenderness.

I am lucky...
I am a survivor,
I am strong,
I am alive and no one can know my pain.

By Angela Steer

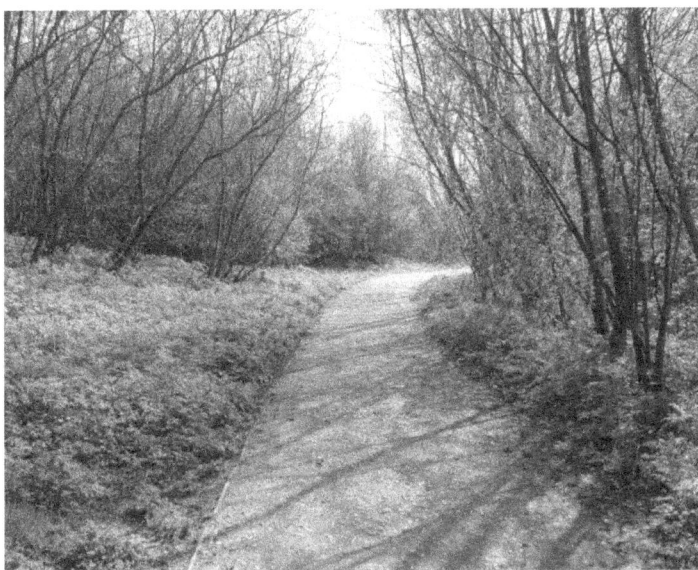

"I'm embracing life, no more wrapping myself up into a silent world and getting depressed. I'm loving life instead of dreading tomorrow."

Wendy Johnson

Reaching for something better

Even though the way is painful & challenging

Choosing more for ourselves than we currently have

Our journey is full of twists and turns

Voicing the past so that we can have the future

Enduring the battles and living for the victory

Remember how far we have come already

Yours is the hope of RECOVERY.

Kate Swift

All I can do is just be Me

When I don't know which way to turn

All I can do is just be me

When I don't know what will happen next, all I can do is just be me

When I want to cry or laugh, sing or shout

All I can do is just be me

When I want to flee or fly all I can do is just be me

All I ever need to do is just BE

By Tasha

R.S.O.S.A

If You Were My Child

A mother's message

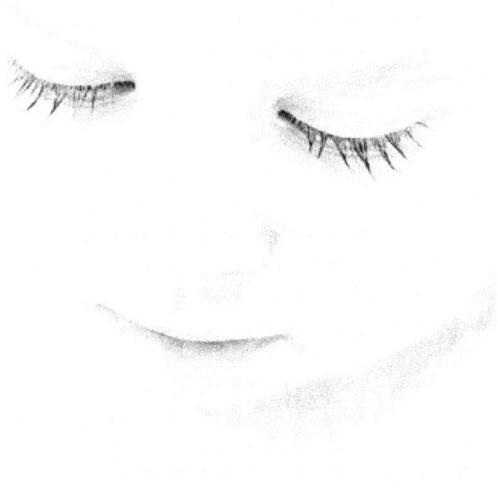

If you were my child I would love you
&
If you were my child I would listen when you
speak and more importantly I will hear you

If you were my child I would look when you ask and
I would see and share your vision
&
If you were my child I would promise to protect
You, but you must trust I know what is best for
your wellbeing

If you were my child your opinions would matter
&
If you were my child I would raise you with
respect and humility

If you were my child you would know right from
wrong

If you were my child I would defend you always
&
If you were my child I would accept you are not
perfect and guide you through your mistakes
If you were my child I would give you
understanding

&
If you were my child I would give you comfort

If you were my child you would grow of the belief
that all things are possible
&
If you were my child your life would come before
all others

If you were my child your life would have
Purpose

If you were my child you would grow with
Encouragement

If you were my child my mistakes would be your
Teacher

If you were my child I would give you all of what
is good and shelter you where possible from harm
and from evil

If you were my child I would teach you to forgive

If you were my child I would teach you loyalty
and honour

If you were my child I would let your journey be
steeped in happiness and learning

If you were my child I would teach you that being

happy with who you are is the most important
attribute you can have

If you were my child I would remind you to
always stand firm in your beliefs

If you were my child I would share the way of the
world with you

If you were my child I would teach you never to
Judge

If you were my child I would teach you the art of
Giving

If you were my child I would encourage kindness
as the best way to proceed

If you were my child I would raise you to think
before you speak

If you were my child I would guide you through
the pathways of truth

If you were my child I would stand in the rain
and dance just because I can

If you were my child my advice would be to
spread your wings and fly free

If you were my child I would educate you to take
your place in the world

If you were my child I would introduce you to the
sun and the sand, the rain and the snow, and
remind you to embrace each season

If you were my child I would raise you to never
take for granted was is real

If you were my child I would instill in you the
value of your worth

If you were my child I would remind you there is
no greater gift than that of self

If you were my child I would remind you to learn
to love self before all others; for without love of
self, love for others is incomplete

If you were my child I would give you the right of
Humanity

If you were my child your life would come before
all others

If you were my child your wrongs I would always
be here to make right

If you were my child your world would be in
colour

If you were my child your heart would know
music

If you were my child your soul would know
Happiness

If you were my child I would raise you with the
knowledge that your mind, your body your spirit
and your dignity are priceless

If you were my child I would remind you to always know your greatest wealth is within the essence of your being; it comes from being able to love and be loved unconditionally; never to be confused with material wealth as it can be here today, gone tomorrow wealth

If you were my child I would raise you to know your home is where love and hope resides; not within the building you lay your head at night

If you were my child you would forever know your home is wherever I may be;
You are as a part of me, as I am of you; let it matter not the dwelling;

If you were my child I would love and protect You

To children the world over this is your right: to grow with peace and with hope; it is your right to have love and light;
Please believe all things are possible!!

We all should be responsible for the children of the world; for their hearts, their minds, their bodies and their souls.

Join me and make children your priority and keep a watchful eye over all children.

Kazzie Kennedy
www.kazziekbooks.com

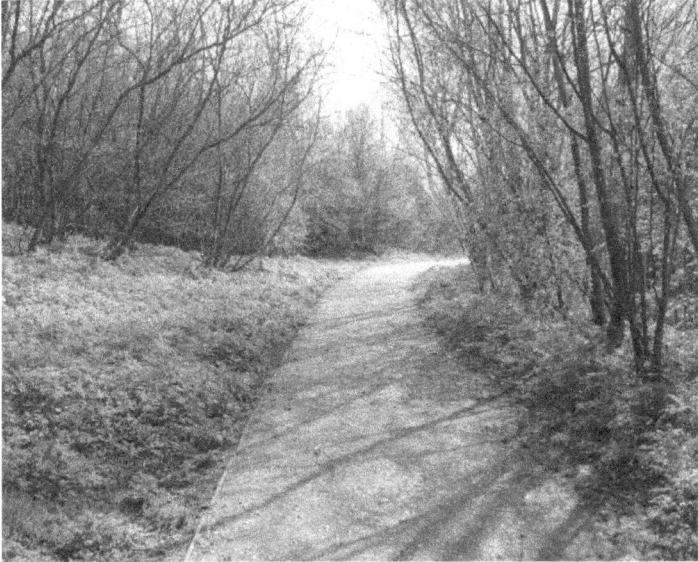

"Do not see yourself as those who have abused you see you, as an object to be taken and used. But rather know that you all are beautiful souls, and that your inner beauty can never be erased by the tragic events that you have had to live through. Prove all those that have abused you wrong and live... live full and fruitful lives"

Ray Redner

FREEDOM

F- free to make my own choices in life.
R- rid all the evil from my life.
E- enjoy my life as it is now.
E- empty out the past and move forward.
D- devote myself to helping others.
O- only look at what Is important and walk away from the rest.
M- my life is worth fighting for.

Mary Calvin

The Peach Tree

When I was a young girl there was nowhere to run to for safety and nobody who ever rescued me. There was just one place where I had a secret sanctuary - the peach tree in my family garden. I made my own little garden under it and decorated it with pretty stones, feathers, anything sparkly, and on extra sad days I'd add one of my special beads. Under the peach tree's safe branches I buried anything that I found dead, birds, insects, and flowers. In my innocence I knew they would be floating to a better world, just like I had longed to do the same.

Here is a page from my healing journal, which documents my journey in drawings and collage...

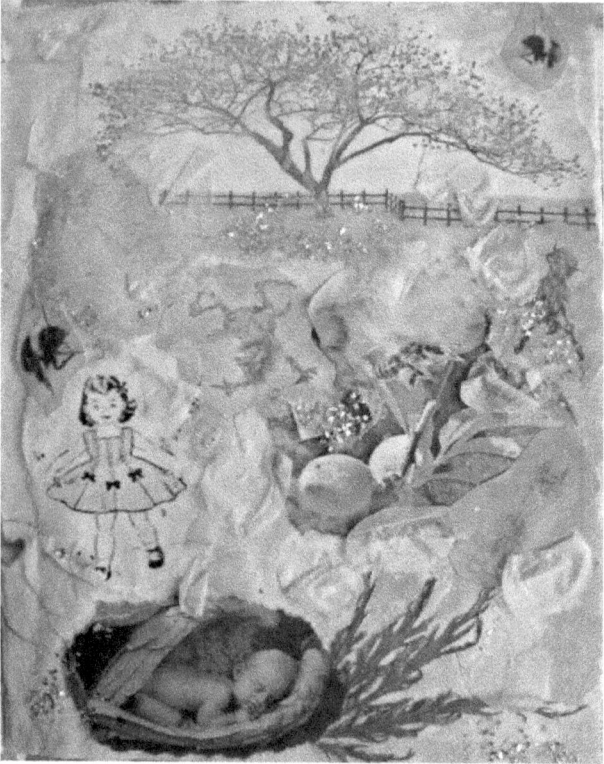

It describes how I was dressed up to look cute - ready to be abused - and all I wanted was to be snuggled up back in the womb - to never come out again. However, for many years, the peach tree was my only real friend. I saw faeries there and maintained my connection to the spirit worlds, which helped to keep me alive. This picture reminds me how I would sit under the tree when the petals were blowing in a warm summer breeze and I'd giggle with delight as the soft pink snow settled on me.

Meryl Aves

God Built My Character

Growing up means different things to each of us perhaps. For some of us, there are more fond memories than bad; for some of us, like myself, the other is true. For me, growing up included being the "shameful, guilty, worthless little girl", always trying to please another, to be accepted and being an easy target. My vulnerability and low self-esteem and the need to feel loved made me a delightful target for an evil molester. Looking back, I have learned to consider the tough times as part of what has made me who I am. And I have credited God for letting me go through even the most difficult times, because I know who I am, I am proud of who I have become and I have seen what others have become.

Character is said to be built, and there is good reason for that. Character does not come easy or cheap. It is nurtured over time, and often involves many tough times and hard lessons. When I was young, I used to ask, "Why?" And with regard to life today, I still sometimes ask "WHY?" The tough times still come, but I always find the heavy doors open easily when I put my trust in GOD.

Knowing that doesn't make dealing with everything a piece of cake, but it sure makes it easier to remember that God is still God, good can come from bad, and I can, in the midst of a storm, still experience His peace. God leads me on a journey today that will turn all my bad into something good. As this good is for others not just myself and that is God's Will, to do good for others. I stand tall today being held in God's arms as I take my ugly past and try to make a beautiful safer future for others.

I admit there will always be plenty of character needing to be built within me, but I am so proud of the character I carry today that has allowed me to reach out to others to help in their healing journeys of abuse and injustice of all types.

Patty Rase Hobson

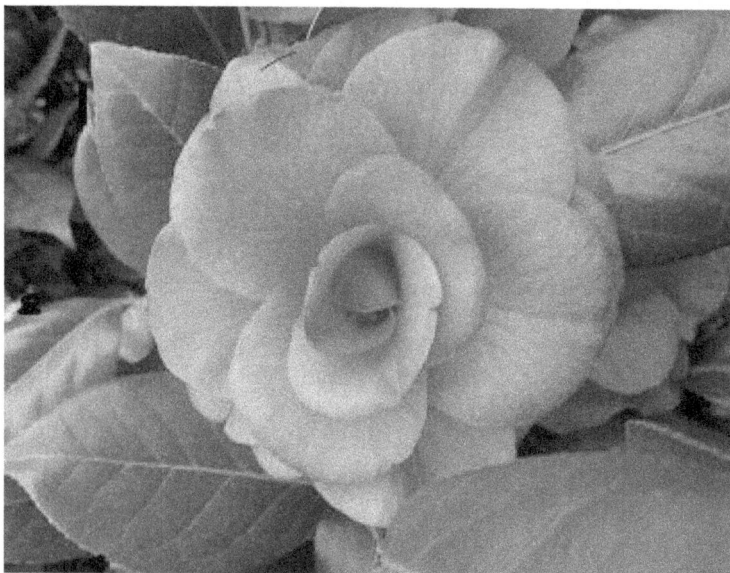

"Always remember, something as simple as planting a tiny seed... can grow into a huge beautiful difference."

Photograph and words by Patty Rase Hobson

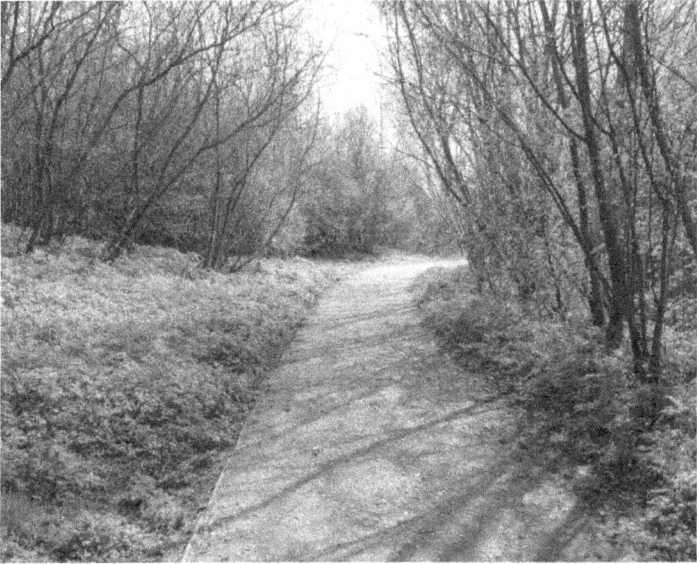

"Looking forward to the day when I can run, well more like fly in my case, across a field screaming "Freedom!!" Someday soon I will have it... and I can't wait. I will get through this."

Sarah Finn

Therapist No. 14

Peter saved me, gave me life; helped me find me.

Kind Peter gave huge time, empathy, sympathy, motivation. He listened; he truly listened to me, like nobody had. One day, I found trust for him.

Once here, we could work hard; confront the demons, the darkness and self hatred.

Peter supported me, guided me; educated me. I felt blind, scared, unsure of where I came from, who I was, where I was going.

For too long, the sessions were full of fear, tears, pain, sadness, anger - there seemed no end, but I did not stop going. I was determined.

Then, I found I could write; I could actually write my thoughts, feelings & memories on paper - the paralysis was no more, I was connecting with me, my soul & facing the fears head on now.

Peter never broke my trust. He wanted to help me. I wanted to change. I spoke freely for the first time to him, I found sound; my voice. I could now share my pain, my shame.

For the first time I saw her; me - the little girl, aged 9, in her bedroom. We hugged, she needed it so. We both did, we both do.

And one day, I could see light, I could see life. Peter was excited with me. I felt I'd been 'away' for years & now I was back on earth: everything was new to my eyes & my senses. It was almost overwhelming & it created a new panic. We continued to work, to confront & to practice using my newly acquired skills.

It was the right time. Peter & I agreed to say goodbye. I was scared but excited too. I felt well equipped for my forward journey... My life.

Since, there have been ups & downs, I think there always will be, but I feel different & I have coped well - with my learned skills which I will always have. My eternal thanks to Peter & to Greg, my GP, for identifying my need & for ensuring I was given such help.

Cecilia

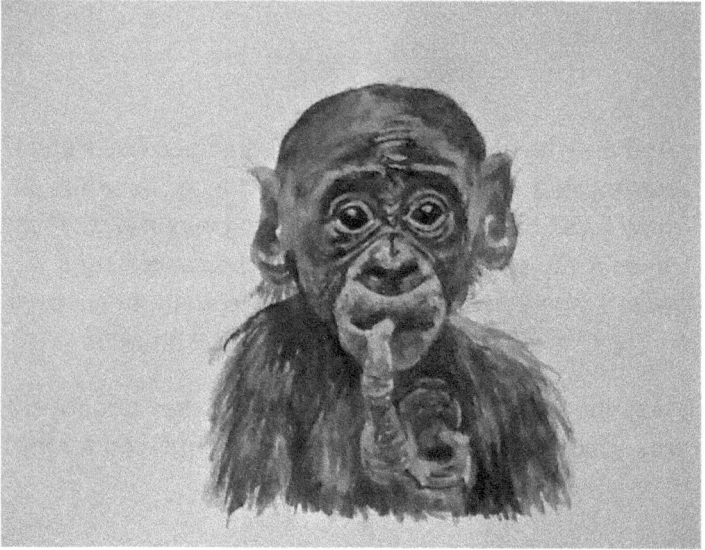

'Oooops! Did I really just say that?'

Wren Murray

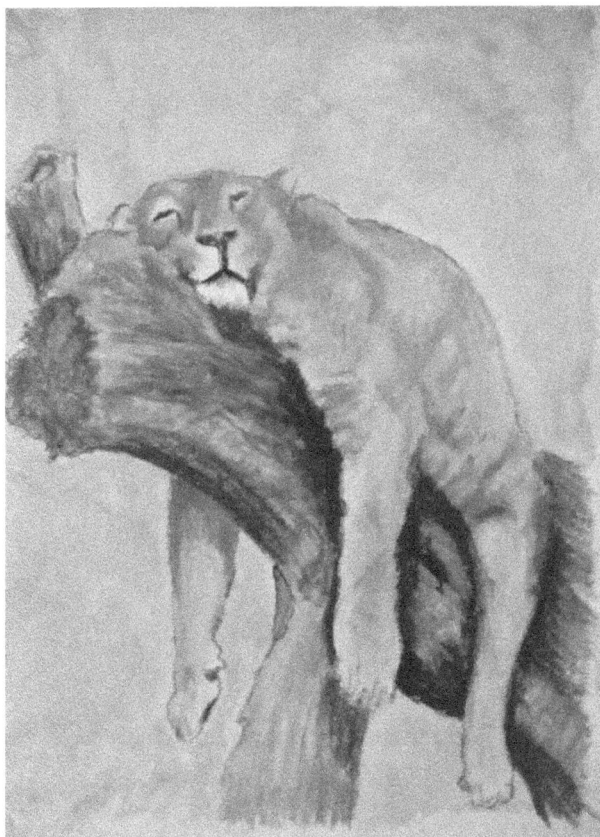

'Me time'

Wren Murray

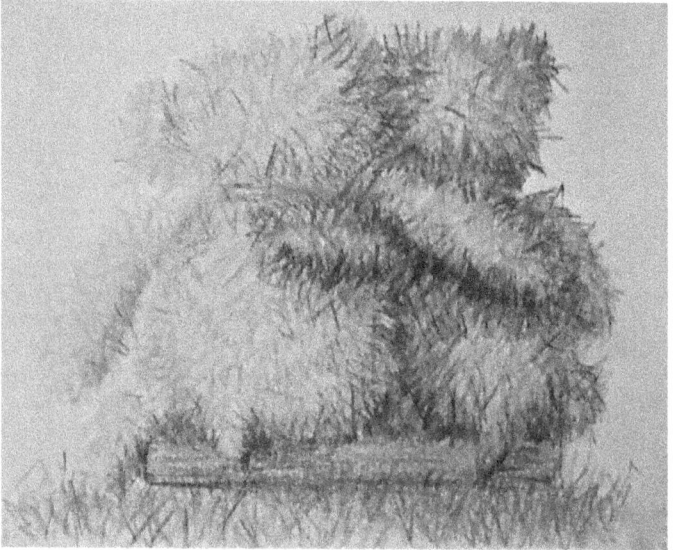

'Teddies know how to hug back'

Wren Murray

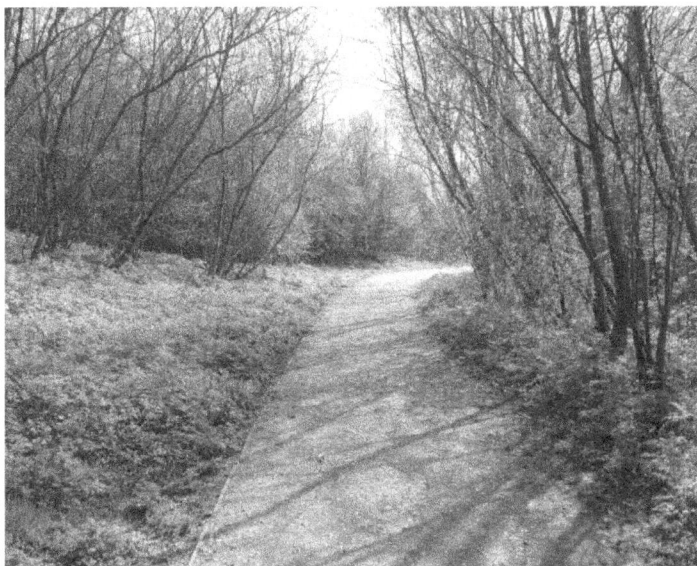

"Sometimes you have to be SO single minded and let nothing de-rail you from what you need to do for you... to bring you to a better place of understanding or of peace for your own life... that is not selfish... it is from time to time *essential* for your own well being & forward journey."

Anon

Growing Up

Growing up is something we all must do; all living creatures grow up. Real growth takes place when things are in tatters. How you cope with the stress is what really matters. You are going to get hurt; the best you can do is get ready for it and even though it hurts at the time; the experience from it will make you stronger. Life always moves on, full stop, no matter what you've lost, or suffered. Everybody else has feelings too; and thoughts racing through their mind on sleepless nights. We all are at our different stages of growing, and we never stop until our earthly eyes close. My wings are still growing, I'm learning something every day; we all are. Making mistakes and growing wiser from them, learning from friends and learning what not to do. Don't try to fight and rush growing up because it'll happen soon enough. You just take have to take it all one step at a time and walk along your road. One step will become two on the path of growth that sometimes is filled with bumps and fast swerves; but in the end you'll see it like a bright shining light... that moment where you realize that you did alright. I've been growing up and I've come a long way. It's been hard, don't get me wrong... I am not done, still have a long way to go... but I am stronger now; I am not the girl I used to be. Growing up is about, learning, discovering, feeling; it's about finding out who you really are and not letting hard times stop you, but embracing them, learning and growing from them. Growing up isn't always easy, we carry all these memories, so many filled with anxieties & worries. We worry far too much, and maybe we should get in touch, with our childhood feelings more. Seasons seem to pass quicker as you grow older, our childhood days, seem so far away...although the memories are never ever gone. There's a time in our lives, where we have to grow up & mature. Growing up opens your eyes to harsh realities that life has to bring and has to offer, but at the same time, it also opens your eyes to the things that really matter and things that you should be most thankful for. Growing up is not easy, just as a lot of things in life are not easy. But once you get the hang of it, it will be the best experience and the best time of your life time. Growing up is a milestone in a person's life that should not be treated lightly. Growing up means you are taking more responsibilities and means that you have to stand your ground on things you believe and principles that dictate your actions.

Sarah Finn

Take a look

Take a look at the world around you. Look at the dark green leaves of the forest during summertime, look at the vibrant colourful flowers blooming in the springtime, look at the pure white snow on the ground; there is such beauty in God's creation; just the little things in your life that bring you joy and excite you. Are they physical things that can easily be thrown away in the garbage or are they things that last longer than physical belongings such as loyalty, truth, friendship, love, honour? Which is more important to you? When life's difficulties frustrate you, take a walk outside, just a short walk, or even just step outside onto your porch and look at the birds flying in the sky, or the snow falling, and really think about what matters to you. Through the past few months, I am learning so much about life, what really matters, how to react to difficult times; and it is honestly an amazing feeling. To finally start to understand the loveliness in such small things; just takes a little time and some patience on your part; take a notebook on what you see, and also what you feel; and you will feel as I am starting to feel, I promise you that you won't forget it.

Sarah Finn

The Young Woman under the Maple Tree

Wandering down a dirt trail deep in the dense forest, your gaze drifts toward a great cherry red maple tree. You notice a young woman sitting against the massive tree trunk, clutching a notebook to her chest, her watchful eye gaping at the multicolored sunset, a lively smile emanating from her face. She's contemplating many things: wondering about where her place is in this world, grappling with her dark habits attempting to exchange them with respectable worthy ones. She has gone through various trials, not always reacting the right way; but that was before she met people, who guided her to start off on the right path. She isn't near her goal, but she knows that she will get through it, no matter what. She knows she is a strong person and had just needed a push. Your face beams at her sunny smile; and you utter a hushed prayer, praying for her to maintain her positive outlook; and you perceive that she will achieve her goal.

Sarah Finn

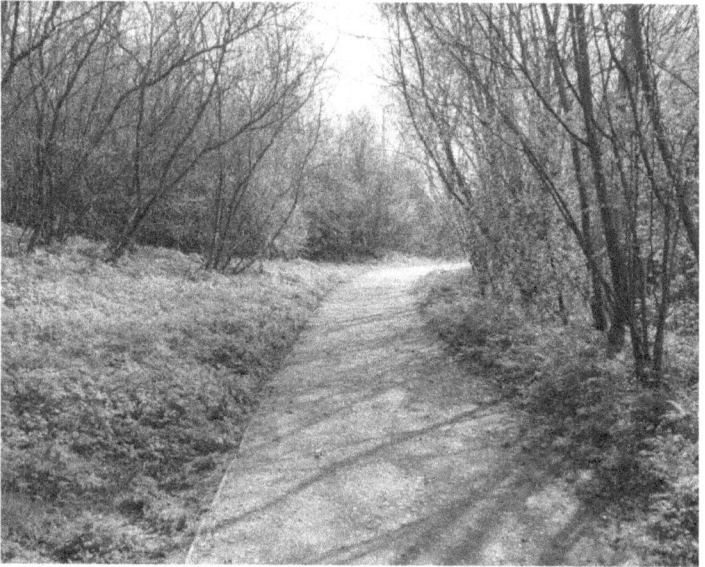

"Every tomorrow has two handles. We can take hold of it by the handle of anxiety, or by the handle of faith."

Author unknown

I didn't realize that the reason I continued to struggle was because I was looking for my answers in all the wrong places. I was searching for an easier way to do the hard work of emotional healing. I wanted someone to tell me what was "wrong" with me - then I wanted them to fix me. I read books thinking "Of so-and-so read this..." instead of reading for my own lessons. When I'd come to the end and had no more options, I realized that the problem wasn't me... that I wasn't broken, didn't need fixing, but that I needed to take all the lessons I'd learned for everyone else and learn how to live for myself.

Susan Kingsley Smith

For many years I believed with all my heart and being that I was broken beyond repair; I believed that the disaster my life was, was my "fault". That I was all the things I was told I was; that I was "bad", "no good"; that I "deserved to suffer"; that no matter what I did it was never "good enough"; that I was not "enough". I began to see that reason was not that I was defective but that those charged with taking care of me horribly violated my trust and taught me to see myself through their eyes as "less than" "worthless" and "unworthy" by the way they spoke to me, the way they looked at me, the way they treated me. Those who were my "mirror" in my youth showed me that I was so horrible and defective that I deserved all the bad things that happened to me; they taught me that I was powerless over myself and my life. They taught me to tolerate the intolerable. Once I started seeing that I wasn't broken but had been taught to see myself through their eyes and their lies, I began to put the pieces of this broken mirror back together. In time I learned to set aside the broken and cracked mirror and I learned to look into a new mirror... the mirror of "me", where I started telling myself that I was not what others said I was, but who I decided to be.

Susan Kingsley Smith

Overcomer

Through the pain,
disappointment,
struggle, I
overcame many
... years of abuse.
The days were
long and hard,
I often wondered
it I would ever
make it.
Lost dreams,
lost hope.
The inner strength,
it came. It dwelled
up in me.
I am a overcomer,
you are too!

Lela Albert

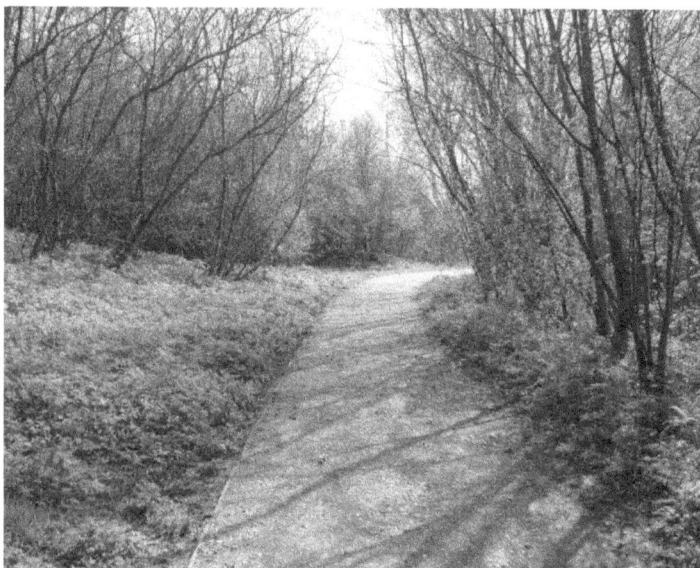

"All of us humans are in search of something, something that can be easily found if you look in the right places and with the right people; and that something is joy."

Sarah Finn

The Free from Addiction Project

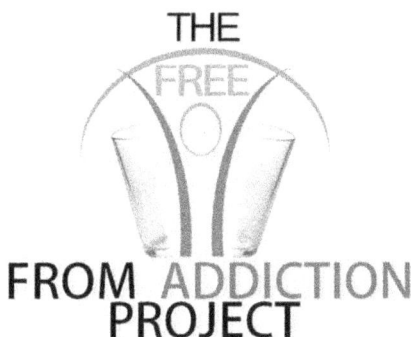

How one man turned his life around

I have faced a lot of obstacles in my life that I have had to overcome and in no way has it been easy. Here are some snippets of my life experiences to date.

My name is Gary Topley, I was born in 1978, in Bedford, and I am one of five siblings. I have two older brothers, an older sister and a younger brother. I was put into care when I was two, as my mum was struggling to bring us all up on her own. She had many difficulties with the problems that she faced, along with the issues that she had surrounding her addiction to alcohol - something that I found later on in my life would affect me too.

~

My first experiences of being in care were at a children's home in Ampthill. After this I went to a foster family in Thurleigh. This was all before the age of four. At four I went to my new family in Dunstable. I always felt I was different in my new family even though I had as much love as and did everything that most children would do throughout their childhood.

~

I had minor brushes with the law for trespassing and shop-lifting, and it seemed to be one thing after another. To top it all off my adopted dad didn't come home that often, or it didn't seem like it. He would spend most of his time in the pub, something that later he would maybe regret, as he also developed an addiction to alcohol. At times I saw him and my mum arguing and, at times, he also showed signs of violence when he was drunk.

~

I moved out of the children's home that I was in and moved into a room in someone's house in Kempston. This again didn't last long: after drinking a bottle of Vodka and a bottle of Bacardi one night I slept in the garage after losing my keys. When I woke up I had never seen such a mess. I walked out of the garage still drunk and saw smashed windows as evidence of how I had tried to get in the house the night before. The landlord was actually quite understanding, but my older brother kept turning up drunk after arguing with his girlfriend and I was eventually told to leave.

I then moved into a bedsit in Bedford. It seemed I had gone full circle, as this is where I was born. The bedsit was in a big house with lots of other bedsits. Drugs and alcohol were rife. I moved between two lots of bedsits, taking amphetamines, drinking, smoking cannabis;I loved my independence.

~

I eventually moved into a hostel. People were in this place for many issues. At first I thought it was okay, but this brought many more problems or, should I say, I created many more. Everyone in there drank, heavily too, and because it had been part of my life previously I started drinking more heavily than I had ever done before, smoking cannabis, fighting and getting arrested. I was seeing my son at this point at a contact centre, but to be honest my life looked bleak and the worst it had done for a long time. While I was at the hostel I started self-harming. I had seen someone else do it at first and I asked him why he did it. He told me it was to get rid of the past and when he saw his arms bleeding he said it was like it was all going away.

~

I was sentenced to Winson Green Prison in Birmingham.

I had never been in prison before so I found it a strange experience. When I first arrived there I was put in a cell that I shared with another man from Melton Mowbray; this was for about a week. I was then moved onto one of the main wings. For what was a short sentence it seemed to drag on forever. One thing I remember is a prison officer saying to me, "Gary, don't spend your life coming in and out of prison. I see it all the time - you have a baby to start thinking about, be there for it." This is something I have always remembered. As daft as it sounds, at the time it didn't make sense, but as time went on it did, more and more. I was released early before the birth of my daughter and put on tag, but to be honest this part of my sentence didn't bother me much because I never really went out anyway. But guess what happened? I started drinking again. I probably was drinking more than I had ever done. 15 pints, 12 bottles of VK and 10 sambuccas was my usual drinking session over about 12 hours. Again, I used any excuse to get out the house and go to the pub. What I did do, though, when I was released was write to the Chief Constable of Derbyshire Constabulary to see if I could do something to help those that had problems with alcohol. I had further meetings with the police and they were sceptical (with every right) as to whether I was serious about changing my life.

~

When I left the Derbyshire Drug and Alcohol Action Team I was involved in other meetings. I thought I would still attend these to try and make a difference, so what I had learned hadn't gone to waste. One meeting I went to, I started talking to someone afterwards. They said to me, "Gary, you have lots of personal experience and know a lot about the alcohol field - Why don't you try and set something up?" I thought she, without being rude, was drunk to be saying that to me - I mean, me, running my own thing to help others. I nonetheless nodded at what I thought was her pie-in-the-sky idea and told her I would. Not having a clue why she said it I went home and sat there in deep thought. "Could I really do something?" "What would it be like?" "What name could I use?" - these questions along with many others were running through my head.

What I managed after a few months, when I had finally made sense of all the questions that I kept asking myself, was to realise that I needed a bit of funding to start everything up. I then went on to spend hours upon hours looking for a place that would give me some initial funding. At times I felt like giving up, but the fact that I had given up on most other things in my life, and my daughter and wanting to do her proud, spurred me on.

Eventually I came across a place so I phoned them, explained what I wanted to do and they sent me an application form to apply for funding to start up what is now known as The Free From Addiction Project.

A month or so went by and I got a letter through the post inviting me in to talk about my visions further, then a couple of weeks later I received a letter saying that my funding application had been accepted. It was only a small amount of funding, a couple of thousand pounds, but it was the start of my new life in doing all I could to help others.

The Free from Addiction project has gone from strength to strength, and has been able to help and support many people battling their own addiction. We also raise public awareness and education about alcohol use and abuse. For more information on what has been achieved, or if you need any help or advice, please visit our website. I also have a facebook page: Gary Topley - Alcohol Awareness Specialist.

Gary Topley

www.freefromaddiction.co.uk

Ready to Shine

When people look at me, what do you they see?

They might see a workaholic girl, a skinny girl that is shy
and timid; or just a not
popular girl.

Now... this is what *I* see in myself:

A girl that is finally starting to come out of the shadows,
ready to show her true self.

One that is...

Not afraid to show herself; one that isn't hiding behind
others

One that is ready to overcome difficulties and hard
times,

A fighter, *not* one that gets defeated easily.

One that is ready to sprout her wings and *shine*.

Sarah Finn

Innocence Betrayed...

I was sexually abused by my stepfather from eight to sixteen. When I was 11 I went to this modeling school. It was run by an elderly man; he had a young girlfriend. I was asked out for dinner one night with them. I was dropped off at his house by my mother. Before we left the lady told me that to be a good model I needed good skin. She got me to take my clothes off, she then rubbed Vaseline intensive care all over my body. They made me feel very special over the weeks, telling me I was going to be a international model. They said they would insure my legs for £10,000 in case they were scarred. They took photos every week. They were grooming me. I was in the top five girls. I did feel very special. After six months I started sleeping there at weekends. There were two other girls too. They started taking nude photos and having sex with us. I never knew it was wrong as my stepfather did similar. When I was 13, the agency closed. My mum told me it was because the man got one girl pregnant. My stepfather would not let the police interview me. The police kept all the really rude photos. This has left me with a lot of problems, mentally and emotionally.

Previously published in *Silent No More*
Re-printed here to give the 2nd piece of writing its context

Reclaiming Some Power

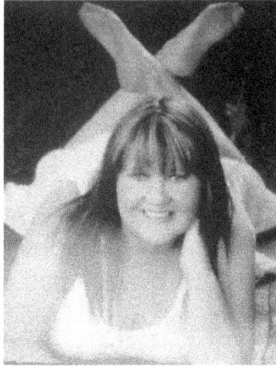

My recovery journey has been long and winding. My sexual abuse was from 8 to 16 (as described above). I started having therapy at 25. I am now 48 and I still see someone. I am feeling a lot stronger these days. I will share a recovery story of mine where I felt I got some of my power back. Being abused has caused some sexual problems for me. Three years ago I got the courage to go to an adult-themed exhibition/show. It was amazing to see everyone not being shy around sex. I now see sex as normal life and not dirty. One of my abusers was from the modelling industry; he took a lot of rude photos of me (under-age). At the exhibition I went to, there was a competition to win a photo shoot, guess what... I won! I was very scared to relive my past in front of the camera but, to my surprise, I was strong and took control of the whole shoot. I feel this has helped my healing. I still get nervous around men but every day I get stronger. I still dream of being a model one day, I live in Victoria, Australia. I guess that makes me a Victoria secret. The photo I have included is from the prize winning shoot I did... and I felt like a princess.

Kerri Nolte

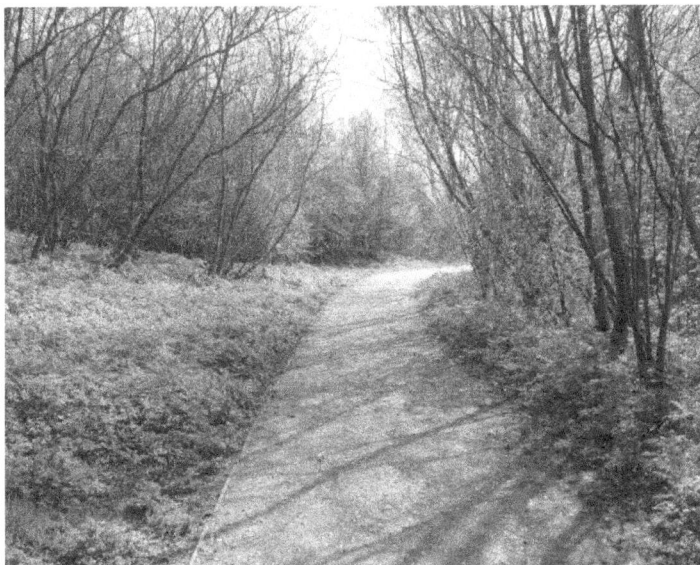

'Remember... Tomorrow is a brand new day.'

Kate Swift

From Devastation to Restoration

It has been a long journey from devastation to restoration, but I've made it to a place where I have nothing to die for and everything to live for. The hardest part of this experience wasn't making the choice to get on the road to restoration... it was the lonely moments deep in the depths of life's depressions that were hardest and that I felt to the marrow of my being.

See... when I was on the road through devastation, it was far from lonely. I had no problem finding people to support my self-destructive ways, but finding people to support me during my heartache, agony and despair; to encourage me to continue forward and to fight for my life? Now that was rare. More often than not my cries were met with resistance and/or discomfort; people sympathized rather than empathized with my circumstances. I found that those who empathized were more eager to mobilize on my behalf and those who sympathized were more likely to send their regards and well wishes. Don't get me wrong, that was nice but it's more like looking at someone with a third-degree burn who is screaming out for help and wishing them well rather than doing *something... anything* on their behalf to either alleviate the pain or supply the resources necessary to aid in the urgency of their need.

Acquiring wellness was not easier said than done, as many imply that it is; however living life in wellness is most certainly easier than living in the exhausting and destructive cycles of devastation. For several years, I had one foot free and one foot embedded in the sludge of existence, living a double life as mother by day and immersed in the world of prostitution by night. This made perfect sense considering I had become a better mother long before I ever became a better woman. The messages I adopted and believed to my core were infectious messages injected by the hands of those who violated me and by the acts of violation themselves. These I took to heart and responded to day in and day out. Hatred, bitterness, resentment for each breath I was compelled to take moment by moment led me to choose to invest in the worthlessness I'd accepted as me.

I was alive to be a mother and in my mind there was nothing after that worth living for, nothing before that worth having lived but for the possibility of them. I wanted with all my being to protect my children from the brutal life I had been exposed to. I wanted to give them a better chance, to show them how to break the cycle and the only way I could do that was to dam that cycle within myself, shielding them from the greatest force of devastation I could expose them to... me. In the process I was slowly imploding and the walls of that internal dam were weakening and I found myself constantly doing damage control.

Eventually, I made a lot of changes, changes as a mother. I taught myself to recondition negative and harmful maternal responses and to supplement my unhealthy impulses with healthier ones. I didn't do it for me, I did it for them. All the while, I was self-destructing as a woman. Who was I? Did I even care? Did I even matter? Would I ever matter? Was I worth discovering? I never saw myself living past the age of 40. Every day I wondered if this would be the day I'd die. Not too often suicidal, but always anticipating the hand of death. I had been convinced it was selfish to think about myself and what I needed so more often than not plowed passed thoughts of wellness.

As is common during the early stages of the process, we find outside reasons to improve our life responses, our children and other loved ones become key influences in our desire for change. Eventually, we may come to the phase where that's no longer good enough... where living through the eyes of others for the prize of their love and acceptance ceases to sustain the cycles of survival. I needed to recondition my total being, mind, body and spirit in favour of me to produce healthier desires.

I was determined to live a contradiction to every mixed, perverted and contaminated message of disgrace and condemnation I'd ever acquired through acts of violation and ignorance. I had arrived at that place where I was consumed by the need to realign my soul. My choice to shift into self consciousness, in the literal sense, caused such an eruption throughout my entire existence that I feared fighting for my own life would cause me to lose my sanity.

There I was, some fourteen years into my adult living experience, deciding to develop a love for self, to live through my own eyes and seek out my own approval. It wasn't too late! I turned a deaf ear to rejection and a blind eye to stigma. I peeled back every available layer of my soul, each fraction and fracture discovered, rediscovered and recovered through knowledge and understanding. I researched myself through deep exploration of my life cycles and development.

I left no reachable stone unturned, processing myself and others by performing 'safety scans' and 'security checks' on my internal and external network. Daily I assessed my responses and that of others towards me. Hyper-vigilance followed by deep decompression sessions led me to eliminate the hate and I began to regulate my responses towards self and others until my old unhealthy responses were no longer my default or reflex response but rather my reflective response. Gratefully, I made it my job to monitor my mind and command my being to come into alignment each morning.

Week by week, month by month and year by year, I affirmed my health and wellness becoming more intimate with my nature as a woman and human being.

An invaluable sense of person grew into an unconditional love of self. I redefined my status in life and terminated my existence. Over time those reflections dissolved themselves out of the equation of choice. I chose me... all of me... and in choosing me I chose better for the lives of those connected to me and manifesting themselves through me.

I gifted *"Rachel"* the grace, mercy and self-compassion I had afforded others and yet deprived myself of. I granted **"Me"** the right to heal... permission to partake in the unlimited power of health and wellness. The mold of destruction in my life had to be broken and a new cast applied. That process alone was in itself a force of great and necessary devastation. My soul was like an uneven side walk not suitable for safe passage and I took a jack hammer to it, crumbling what was left of it. I then took the rubble and recycled it into a new foundation... a new path to journey along. While this path provides a much safer passage through life, the initial process of restoring to a state of wellness was by no means a beautiful experience.

When the conditions are ripe and we are determined to achieve wellness, it is then that we begin to process through the saving grace of restoration. Having lived through the compounding impacts of childhood maltreatment, chronic sexual abuse, domestic violence and medical neglect, I know firsthand that restoration is a lifelong process. However, there is a stage that can be reached where, despite the difficulties of each shift and phase, we naturally become compelled to yield to wellness and a healthier lifestyle is manifested.

Restoration is the result of identifying, establishing, applying and or supplementing healthier behavioral response patterns consciously, consistently and deliberately until naturally. It is the establishment of self-worth and personal value, the realization that we are not alone and to achieve maximum results from this process we must not go it alone. We must network with other violation survivors, share, relate, celebrate, prune and groom one another towards healthier living.

I will never forget my mentors and the love they shared with me. I will forever be grateful to them for their wisdom and the safe direction they guided me towards. Because of them, I have learned how to yield to wisdom, my greatest teacher. This is how we modify soul and manifest a new norm... one worth thriving for.

In the process of establishing my new norm, I acknowledged my life purpose. I will always recall that moment when I realized that everything I had experienced during my days of dependency didn't define me but rather defined my purpose in life. From that moment forward, my life experiences made good sense and I was able to rapidly transform my pains into my gains.

It is my purpose and goal to complete *The Milano Method Book on a Layman's Approach to Human Survival and Restoration.* I also aim to publish accompanying publications and to establish The L.I.G.H.T (The Living Institute of Guidance, Hope and Transformation). These are to be social and environmental tools to facilitate, support and enrich the lives of Violation Survivors globally. I will always be an author and sandartist; this is how I make more to do more with.

Strategically, we can aid in preventing the socio-economic collapse of those struggling through their survival while facilitating the maintenance and application of each individual's will to thrive. It is only through my fumbles that I am able to establish what is required to achieve these goals. I don't know how to do a lot of things but I know how to apply the power of restoration and how to motivate people to get on the journey through healthier living. Yes, this I know very well.

I have discovered a great many things which I will share with all who will hear. Having experienced life's journey through destruction and devastation, I have established that one of my primary missions is to re-educate the general populous on what it means and what it is to be a Violation Survivor and to thrive beyond survival. I established the term *Violation Survivor* because it is the closest to authentically identifying who we are as a collective... *survivors of violation.* Some of us have been raped, some tortured, others beaten, many mentally, emotionally and spiritually abused while others continue to be unlawfully neglected. This is compounded by the social shame and stigma assigned to us by those who promote ignorance over the application of sound knowledge, compassion, mercy and a healthy dose of grace. It has become clear that there is an urgent need to introduce a new vocabulary that is respectful of Violation Survivors worldwide and I will do my part in assuring that transpires.

Over the past five years, I have worked full-time with thousands of Violation Survivors and have heard a unified voice pleading for greater understanding in regards to our circumstances and conditioning. As a result, I have developed phrases and terms to advocate *safer survivor communication.* These are terms created not by mass media and encouraged by propaganda to micro-manage that which they fail to comprehend, but rather terms generated on behalf of those who know all too well what it feels like to be on the receiving end of social, professional or political ignorance and intolerance.

Too many violation survivors run from the seats of therapy for lack of genuine understanding by clinical professionals. Life is not according to the book... the book is according to life and many books have reached their expiration marks and yet those same theories, theologies and beliefs remain applied to the mental health patient. It is time for the clinician and the layman, the professionals and the thriving survivors to unite their expertise for the advancement of all. The season for valuing and incorporating the life lessons gained by thriving survivors is long overdue.

It is my hope that this new language of love and respect promotes freedom of expression amongst Violation Survivors to help us establish a healthy and accurate dialog with those who are unable to relate. There was a time when the mentally challenged demanded they not be called 'retarded' or 'stupid' or 'dumb' and when the gay community demanded proper expression and use of terminology, and taught society what was inappropriate about the words loosely thrown around about them. Compassionless communication always adds insult to injury.

Now is the time to demand the respect and honour we deserve, having endured far too much stigma and dejection as a result of having been violated. Enough acceptance of ignorance and being socially groomed to feel a sense of false guilt with regard to "our role" in violation. Enough being force-fed how we are expected to feel, deal and heal. It is time for us to express and share the reality of being Violation Survivors and introduce our norm to the mainstream declaring that we are no longer subject to assigned shame and fear.

In my years of actively working to re-educate the populous, I get asked a lot of questions. One of the most common is, "Rachel, what is the process?" The process is one of lifestyle transformation. Restoration is not about going back to re-obtain who we were 'meant' to be, but rather growing forward, developing who we are in this moment as survivors and thriving survivors continuously seeking a renewed state of health and wellness. Restoration is about living the healthiest version of 'self' each day in the 'as-is condition' until 'as-will-be' manifests. We do this accompanied by the pains we are consciously, pro-actively and willfully resolving and healing through.

Restoration is where we reach a point of thriving beyond survival while acknowledging we can apply our will to live true to who we are in the moment, according to our unique abilities and capabilities. It is about respecting the journey we have experienced, honouring and appreciating it by processing its' worth in our lives. We obtain restoration by continuously valuing and applying the life lessons we discover and sharing them with all those who are connected to us.

There are several cycle types a victim of violation will go through during the course of life. At the moment of violation, we became victims. Those who do not die are surviving victims. Some victims live in victim mode for quite some time, perhaps years. Others eventually shift destructively towards becoming a victim-abuser, further violating themselves or others in cycles of behavior that risks the health and safety of those they share their lives with. These cycles almost always manifest new victims of violation; often these victims are children and loved ones.

Many victims will shift to the state of a struggling survivor, seeking desperately to go back to being 'normal' by 'getting over it', 'leaving the past in the past', always falling short of feeling, dealing and healing their wounds. Like fish flailing in shallow shores, they soon find these cycles to be life-threatening. Alone in the middle of the night, they weep in agony or succumb to silent addictions to numb away the impulse to touch the pain and to find healthy ways to process it. Soon their lives and the lives of those they care for are overwhelmed by their compulsions, addictions and distractions such as shopping, eating, sex, gambling, substance abuse, victim-ism (those addicted to being a victim) and etcetera. This is a lifestyle ruled by fear and shame.

A vast majority of struggling survivors will shift into survivor recovery, entering programs or developing their own means of recovering from the devastating impacts of violation. For most, this reveals itself over time as an incomplete stage, many believing they have recovered and are well, never quite reaching a point in their lives where they are thriving... suddenly and rudely realizing they are still surviving, triggered and haunted by under recovered wounds. Like a cancer, they come out of remission and old default response patterns surface for crisis management and often times those patterns are unhealthy responses to life.

Then there are those who shift into Restoration, the wide road to living as a thriving survivor, free from the shackles of shame, living stigma free and renewed by the enrichment of each day, living and loving themselves through their established new norm. Incapable of being compelled to respond in the old cycles of destruction, these thriving survivors fully transform from Devastation to Restoration, victoriously emerging as the living miracles they have always been.

I have not only experienced every stage of survival but I have *come through/processed through* every stage of survival. Now, as a thriving survivor of violation I want nothing more than to leave behind a blueprint, a map to the greatest treasure known to mankind, the map to 'soul-self'. I am living the reason I endured, this purpose I've secured, this foundation I thrive upon free of condemnation... I am living in truth, trust and triumph... celebrating my victories because I am capable of being victorious!

So, how long did it take me to go through this process of restoration and wellness?

To that, my long-winded philosophical response remains; this entire living experience has been a process filled with core, surface and subsurface equations, summations, stimulations, evaluations, impulses, types, defaults, determinations, portions, rations, alignments, modifications, observations, lessons, absorptions, saturations, incorporations, participations, hesitations, phases, shifts, waves, stages, levels, frequencies, cycles, rotations, revolutions, revelations, resonations and orbits centerd around circumstantial conditions of perceptual enrichment and or deficiency, all which are ever redefined... purposefully. Therefore, I would say it has taken all my life to experience the cycles of restoration while in contrast it took a good portion of my life to be impacted by and in tune with cycles of devastation.

In short, life has not finished with me yet... it is to be continued and I am honoured by the opportunity to further develop my personal health and wellness. There is so much I could share... volumes that, I'm sure, are to come. However, what I hope is that this small glimpse into how I have become a thriving survivor of sexual abuse, domestic violence, childhood maltreatment and neglect will encourage even a few to embrace the journey through restoration. To inspire them to appreciate its pricelessness.

Remain safe, remain well and may love and life continue within you all. Until next time, look for me... I am emerging in the cycles of life, the space where we discover and develop through devastation and restoration.

Ms Rachel E Milano

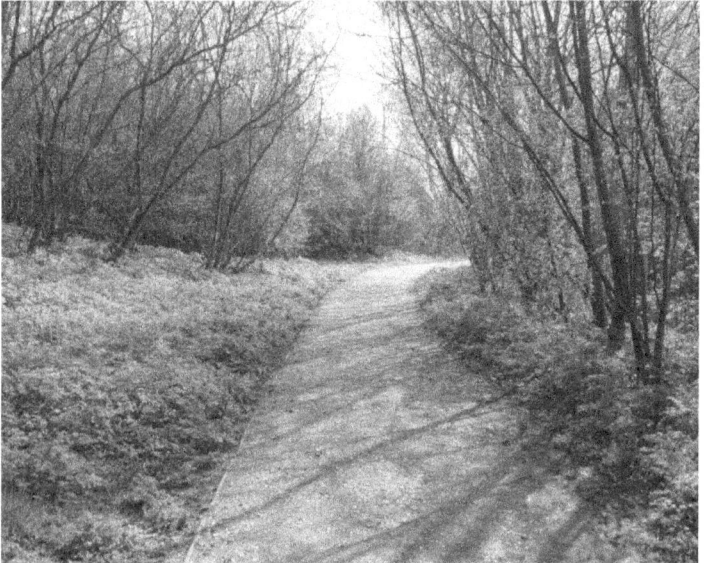

We who are survivors... of which we are many... are in this journey
& this fight for something better - together... you are not alone

Kate Swift

The Child Within

Abused and abandoned
The child within
Suppressed and stunted
The child within
Kept in the dark
The child within
There will be sun and she will win
I will find my child within

Alison Harmer

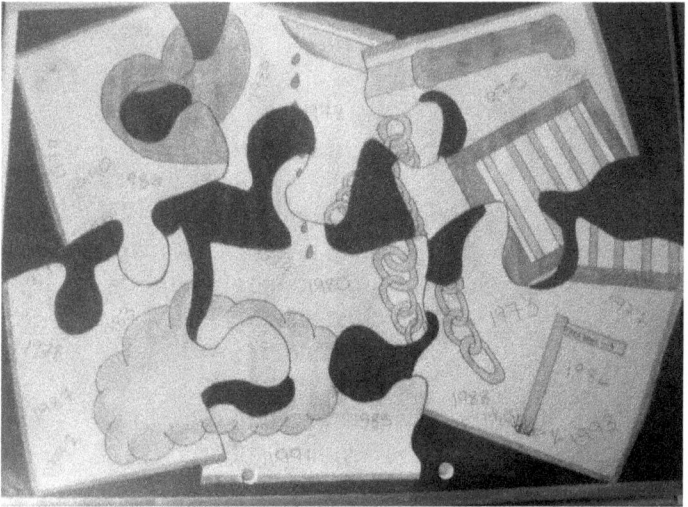

By Jo

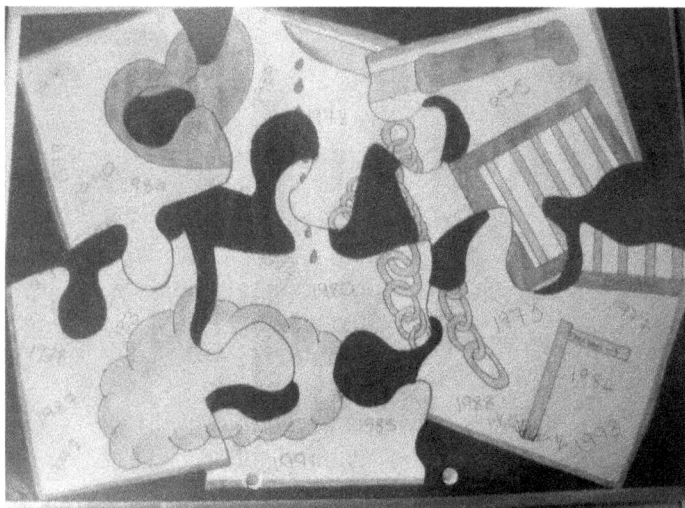

By Jo

Finding Happy Memories

As a survivor I found that by blocking out the bad memories of my past I had also lost anything good. Through therapy I am now able to access and work through the trauma but was finding it difficult to reach the good stuff. I then came across a book about growing up in the 70's and this has been the key to remembering happier times. Suddenly I was thinking about all the great tv programmes I had watched as a child. The book also talked about all the toys that had been available back then. It was like turning back the clock but separating out the good bits. These are the memories that I want to keep in my head. Eventually the bad stuff will hopefully be sorted out and stored away. But I will hold on to the good memories and when I think about playing on my space hopper I will smile.

Jo R

Silent Too Long

I speak for those whose smiles are hiding
The hurt that is beyond confiding

I speak for the wife--the girlfriend
Bearing bruises from the men they defend

I speak for the confused, adolescent boy
Who has somehow become the coach's toy

I speak for those whom no one sees
For those who feel they are diseased

I speak for those whose tongues are stilled
For those with no hope of ever being healed

I speak for those who have endured unspeakable things
For those who never see the hope that dawn brings

I speak for those who have no voice
For tiny babies never given a choice

I speak for those whose lives are living hell
For those wishing they had someone to tell

I speak for those with innocence taken
Who pray for the day they never awaken

I speak for you whose spirits have flown
To let you know--you are not alone

I speak for you, I feel your pain
I will not be silent while evils remain

I speak for you and-- I speak for me
I speak for the world to hear and see

I speak for those with no will to fight
To bring the secrets and darkness to light

I speak because I was silent too long
I speak because I did no wrong

I speak though there are those who would silence me
I speak because abuse should never be allowed to 'be'

Penny Smith

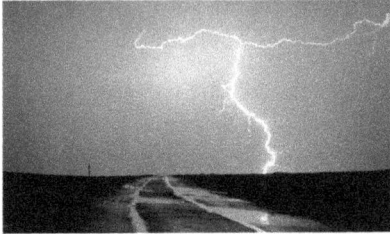

We Thunder

I was the thunder and the thunder was me
We raged and roared in the heavens
In a tear-slinging symphony
Washing away the badness and sadness
We sung our song together
In harmony
What a release…
To feel ALIVE
I feel strong like the thunder

Angelite

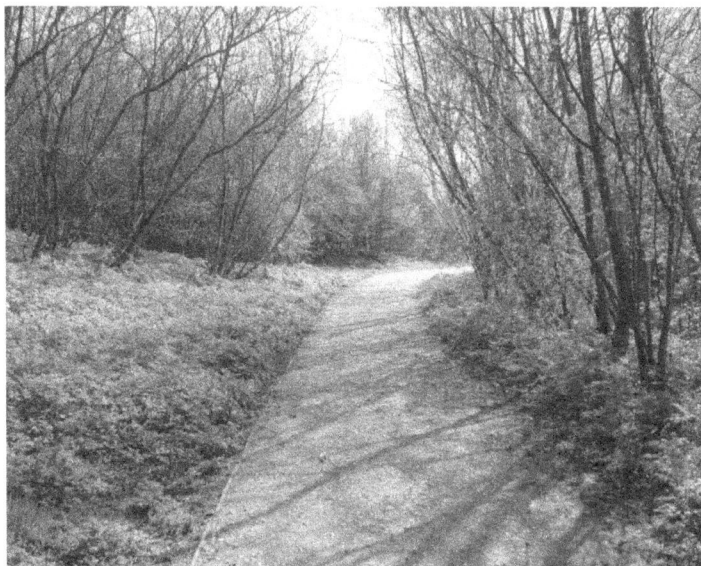

"I never thought I would ever have a day when I would be free of thoughts of self-destruction. It goes to show that when you work to free yourself of what hurts and eats you inside, it will change all your thoughts about life. So amazing!"

Alison Harmer

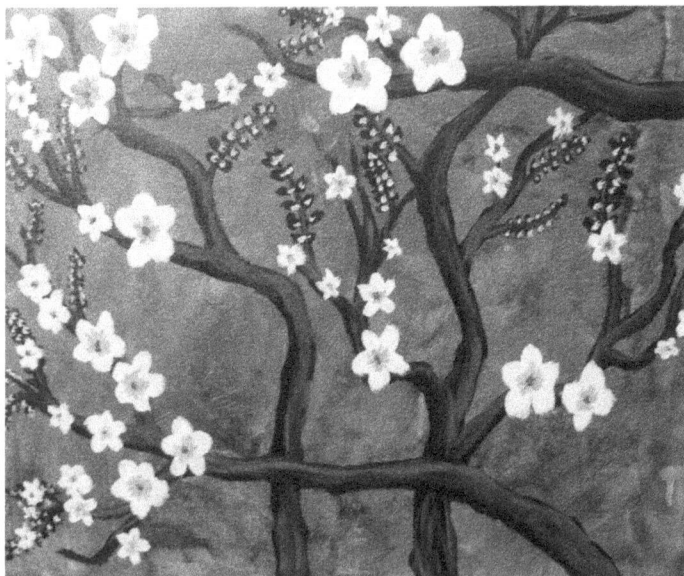

Jess Reece

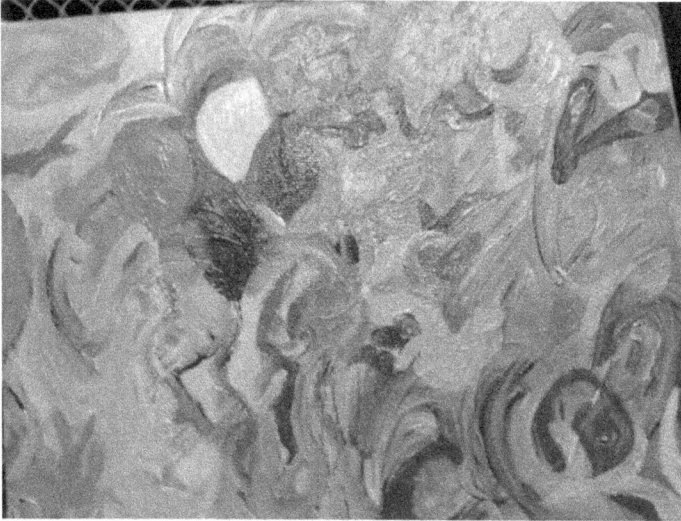

'Underneath the pain and mess there is a party to be had.'

Kerri Nolte

Spring

Spring has sprung
With blossom on trees

Spring has sprung
With March madness

Spring has sprung
With April showers

Spring has sprung
With May fairs

Spring has sprung
With new life

Spring has sprung
With new hope

Ed Shearer

Acorn

I am an acorn
Hard on the outside
Waiting to grow
Needing to break free

I am an acorn
Breaking the shell
Dying to my self
So I can break free

I am an acorn
In the ground
I have shed my shell
I am breaking free

I am an acorn

Ed Shearer

Walls

Today my walls came crashing down
The walls that made me frown
Maybe tomorrow I'll smile
Just for a while

When they crashed
I thought my hopes were dashed
Tomorrow I'll smile
Just for a while

When I let you in
I can't hear the din
Today I'll smile

Yes smile
Just for a while.

Ed Shearer

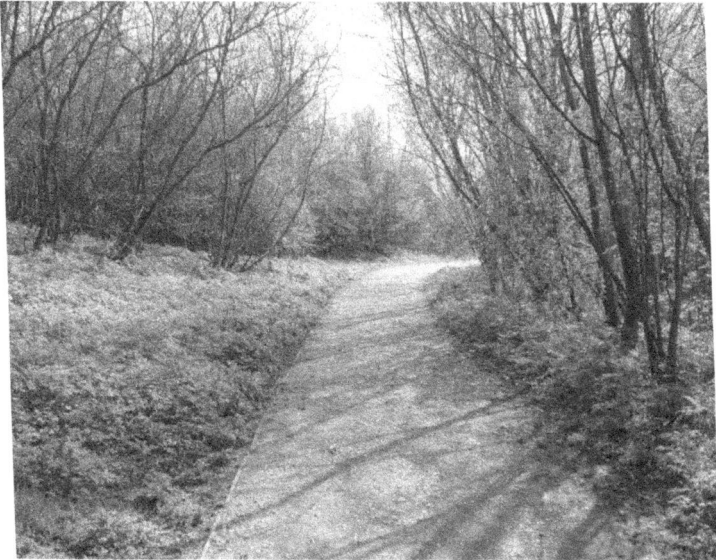

'Tomorrow is yours to shape and mould into what you
want it to be.'

Anon

Our 'Survivor Coffee Morning' Art Project

'For years we have filled the boxes in our minds with sadness and pain, now we take control by creating a box full of happiness and positivity.'

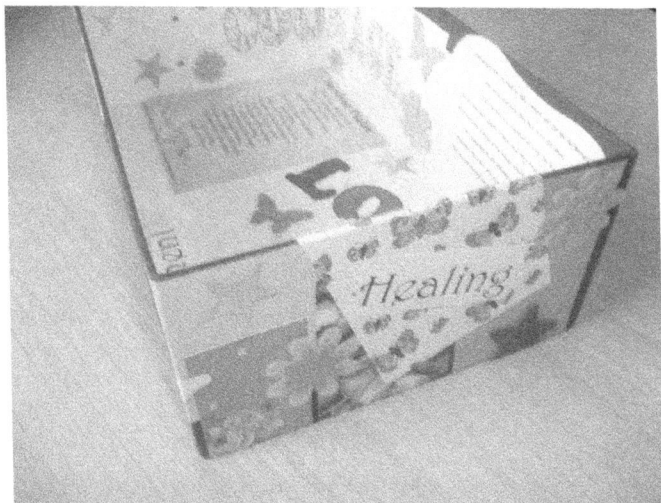

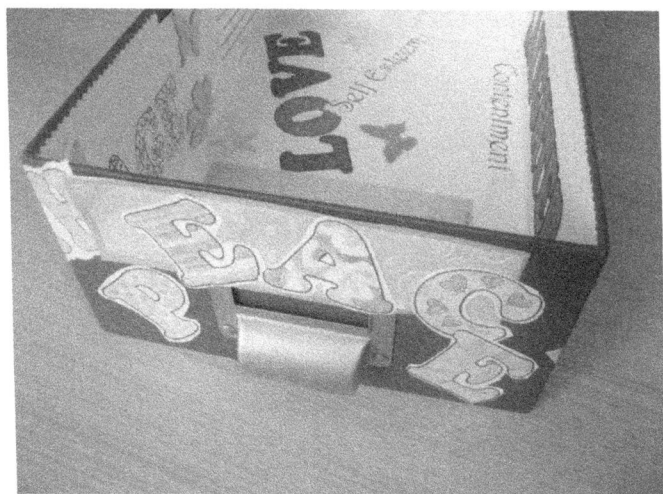

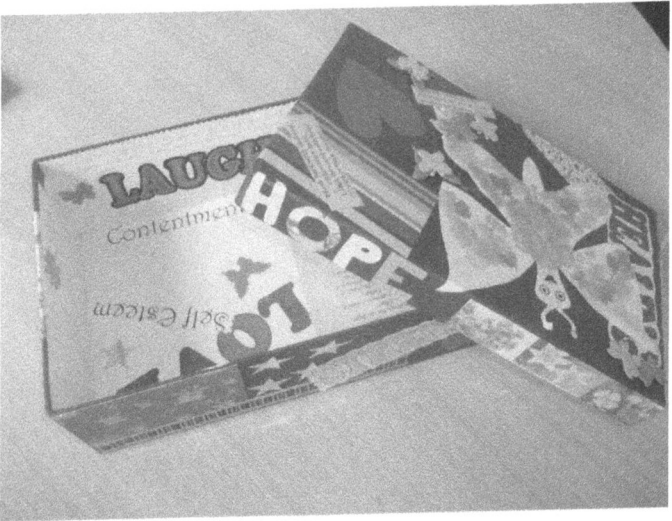

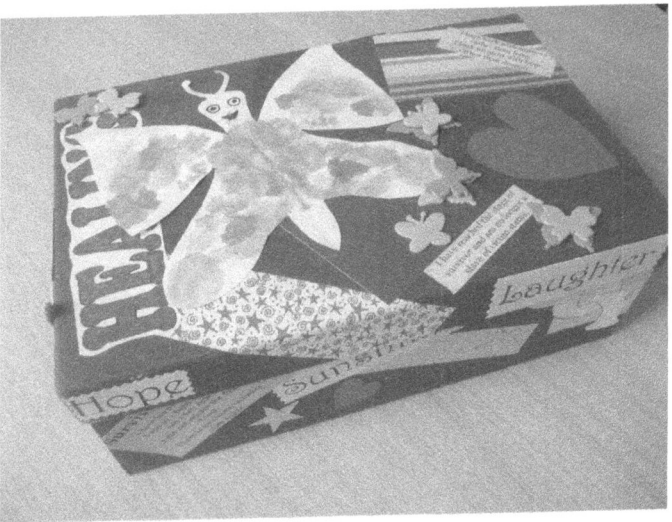

By T.T.W Survivor Coffee Morning Group

Jo – Lorraine Hawkins – Natasha – Fru Hayler – Amy – Kate Swift

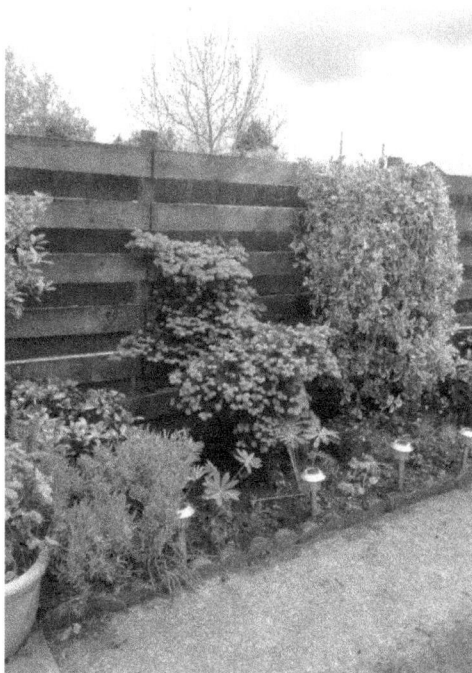

Time to Blossom

I have asked those who have supported me through my path to healing to suggest plants for my garden. I have chosen as near as I can to what everyone has suggested. I have lilies, roses, lavender and herbs, and will get snow drops in the autumn to plant up for next year. My garden is filled with love that will bloom. After all, it is the love of those that have helped me to blossom.

Alison Harmer

* 9 7 8 1 8 4 9 9 1 8 7 6 3 *